Multidisciplinary Management of Chronic Pain

Sridhar Vasudevan

Multidisciplinary Management of Chronic Pain

A Practical Guide for Clinicians

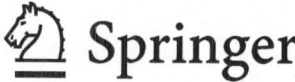 Springer

Sridhar Vasudevan
Wisconsin Rehabilitation Medicine Professionals
Milwaukee, WI, USA

ISBN 978-3-319-36171-0   ISBN 978-3-319-20322-5   (eBook)
DOI 10.1007/978-3-319-20322-5

Springer Cham Heidelberg New York Dordrecht London
© Springer International Publishing Switzerland 2015
Softcover reprint of the hardcover 1st edition 2015

Printed on acid-free paper

Springer International Publishing AG Switzerland is part of Springer Science+Business Media
(www.springer.com)

This book is dedicated to Joyce Anne Vasudevan, my best friend, mentor, and supportive wife

Foreword

Twenty-odd years ago, Dr. Sridhar Vasudevan prepared an outstanding and well-received guide for patients with chronic pain. By the time that valuable overview appeared, Dr. Vasudevan was already regarded as a master clinician whose empathy, ability to motivate patients through recovery, and knack for distilling complex phenomena into simple, striking metaphors was widely acclaimed. Since then, Dr. Vasudevan has continued his string of accomplishments and service not only to patients with pain and their loved ones, but also to the broad community of health care professionals involved in their care. This latter service has ranged from the presidency of the American Academy of Pain Medicine (AAPM), an organization founded by pain physicians, to multiple professional and patient-centered leadership roles.

During the past decade, many members of the pain community and organizations such as AAPM have recognized the huge social and economic burden of pain and the need for education of frontline practitioners about it. Primary care is where the majority of pain problems are seen and treated—ideally, with sufficient expertise and promptness to avoid their evolving into disabling, demeaning (and stigmatized) chronic pain. In this concise yet comprehensive gem of a volume, Sri Vasudevan has combined a summary of the specialist pain literature with personal insight and expertise, including his own metaphors that he uses to explain in a reassuring, even therapeutic fashion many clinical aspects of pain.

I believe this guide will be read and used as a resource not only by health care providers, but also by those patients and their families who want to delve deeper into a current, well-informed understanding of their condition and to support self-management whenever possible. As president-elect of AAPM, I am proud to count Sri Vasudevan among the ranks of its outstanding leaders and role models.

Daniel B. Carr, MD, DABPM, FFPMANZCA (Hon)
Director, Program on Pain Research, Education and Policy
Professor of Public Health (Primary), Anesthesiology and Medicine (Secondary)
Tufts University School of Medicine, Boston, MA, USA
President-Elect
American Academy of Pain Medicine

Foreword

For over 20 years, I was involved in a multidisciplinary chronic pain treatment team at a major academic hospital. As one of the leading programs in the country, we had frequent visits from health professionals from around the world. Many were practitioners who were familiar with multidisciplinary pain treatment but wanted to learn much more about the practical aspects of evaluating and treating patients with complex, chronic pain problems. Invariably, a visitor would ask, "Why don't you write a practical guide to multidisciplinary pain treatment that includes all the tips and suggestions you've shared with us?" At the time, we were focused more on publishing rigorous research studies, an effort that eventually led to my publishing over 300 papers on pain assessment and treatment. The book, unfortunately, never was written.

At present, the need for practical information for clinicians managing chronic pain has never been greater. Chronic pain has reached epidemic proportions with yearly costs exceeding those of heart disease and cancer combined. Well-intentioned efforts to manage chronic pain by liberalizing the use of opioids has have disastrous consequences in the USA in that it has been accompanied by a significant rise in opioid-related deaths and disability. Although injections and surgery have helped some patients with chronic pain in the short run, their effectiveness in the long run is increasingly questioned. To make matters worse, in the past 10 years many established multidisciplinary pain programs in the USA have been closed or downsized. As a result, most patients with entrenched and complex problems coping with pain are now being treated in the primary care setting. There is growing recognition among primary care doctors of the limitations of their traditional approaches to medically treating these patients and heightened interest in multidisciplinary approaches that can be integrated into the primary care setting.

Over the course of a long career, Sridhar Vasudevan has had a rich set of experiences in multidisciplinary pain management. He has been involved in providing pain rehabilitation services since 1973 and has treated thousands of patients suffering from chronic pain. Furthermore, as director of a pain clinic for 10 years and then as medical director of a comprehensive pain program for more than 27 years, he is intimately familiar with how to integrate the expertise of professionals from multiple disciplines so as to meet the unique needs of a given patient. I first met Dr. Vasudevan at major pain research meetings held in the USA and abroad where he was actively involved in both giving and attending presentations. In many ways, he has always struck me as the embodiment of the scientist-practitioner, i.e., one who not only can understand and incorporate scientific advances into his practice, but whose clinical experiences inform and shape his own (and others') research.

In this book, Dr. Vasudevan draws upon an accumulated reservoir of clinical expertise to provide readers with an up-to-date and highly readable clinical guide to multidisciplinary pain management. The book provides numerous practical tips and suggestions. These include simple diagrams, analogies, and anecdotes that can be used to help patients understand the complexity of chronic pain. Used as part of a treatment rationale, such approaches can enhance the ability of patients to engage with and follow through with treatment recommendations such as the need to exercise, increase activity level, and use relaxation and other cognitive behavioral approaches. The book addresses controversial issues that primary care physicians struggle with such as the utility of chronic opioid therapy. Concerns related to the increased use of spinal fusions for chronic back pain are highlighted, such as costs, recovery time, and complications. Practitioners in primary care settings will find the chapter on evaluation of disability in patients with chronic pain especially helpful.

One of the most interesting and unique chapters in this book is the one entitled "Creating a Multidisciplinary Team." The chapter chronicles the demise of multidisciplinary programs in the USA, a trend that occurred despite the fact that the evidence base for this approach has never been stronger. Interestingly, because of this evidence base, the multidisciplinary approach is thriving in countries outside the USA. Undaunted by the downturn in funding for multidisciplinary programs, Dr. Vasudevan recently has been teaching health professionals how they can develop their own "virtual" multidisciplinary treatment teams. He draws on that experience in this chapter and provides numerous practical tips for identifying patients most likely to benefit from this approach and for finding professionals in one's local area who are suited to this work. Dr. Vasudevan also addresses key issues such as developing and sustaining cross-disciplinary communication, something critical to treatment success. Practitioners will find his discussion of the roles of key virtual members of a multidisciplinary pain management team (physicians/nurse practitioners, physical therapists, occupational therapists, psychologists/counselors) to be especially helpful.

The virtual multidisciplinary team represents a cost-effective approach to providing high-quality clinical care to patients suffering from chronic pain. It is likely to become widely used in the future. Advances in technology, such as the shared electronic medical record, face-to-face video communication over the Internet, and self-management applications to support pain management, will play an important role in the implementation of such virtual approaches to chronic pain management.

The chapter on "Patient Stories" is intriguing because it makes the multidisciplinary pain management approach come alive. Three detailed case studies are presented, all of which illustrate the tragic history of events that all too often set the stage for chronic pain. Each of these case studies describes the psychological and social devastation that can be wrought by chronic pain. The iatrogenic effects of medical approaches designed to help each patient are nicely illustrated. These case studies strongly show how multidisciplinary treatment approaches can work together to address biological, psychological, and social factors that may be contributing to pain.

Considered overall, this timely and well-written book has much to offer. Because it is loaded with clinical tips, health professionals from all disciplines who work with patients with chronic pain will find it useful. If only this book were available years ago, so that when a visitor to our own program had asked for a practical guide to multidisciplinary pain management we could have handed him this book.

Francis J. Keefe, PhD
Director, Pain Prevention and Treatment Research Program
Professor, Department of Psychiatry and Behavioral Sciences
Professor of Psychology and Neuroscience
Professor in Anesthesiology, Duke University School of Medicine
Durham, NC, USA
Editor-in Chief of PAIN
The Journal of the International Association for the Study of Pain

Foreword

Dr. Vasudevan is a true champion of multidisciplinary pain management, and this book is a testament to his many years of patient care, research, and teaching in this endeavor. His target in this volume is the health care provider who treats chronic pain patients and recognizes that traditional biomedicine does not provide adequate diagnostic or therapeutic tools. After a brief introduction, he first outlines the problem of chronic pain and lays out all the issues. Next is a chapter on the various theories of the mechanisms for chronic pain. Brief presentations of the various explanations for chronic pain are helpful to understand the multidisciplinary approach to chronic pain management. The fourth chapter, written by Drs. Smerz and Grunert, describes cognitive behavioral strategies that are useful in the treatment of patients suffering from chronic pain. The fifth chapter describes many of the treatments aimed at chronic pain patients that have no proven utility for the patient although they may generate significant revenue for the provider.

Chapter 6 is the meat of this book, as it describes how to treat the chronic pain patient with a rehabilitative program that is based upon a biopsychosocial model. All aspects of this therapeutic program are outlined, including the optimal use of pharmacologic agents. The risks of long-term opioid use are thoroughly discussed. The essential principle of this type of treatment is that the patient must do the work to overcome his pain and suffering; health care providers offer guidance, teach skills, and provide support for what is for most patients a difficult journey.

Chapter 7 addresses the evaluation of disability and how the provider should interact with the patient and the disability system. Unfortunately, the latter often undermines rehabilitative treatments for chronic pain patients. Chapter 8 is important, as Dr. Vasudevan addresses the often thorny issue of creating and maintaining an interdisciplinary team for patient management. Chapters 9 and 10 address some of the common chronic pain diagnoses: low back pain, fibromyalgia, myofascial pain syndromes, and complex regional pain syndromes. Several patient stories precede the concluding chapter, which summarizes the key points presented in the prior chapters. Clinical pearls that are derived from the author's personal experiences are found in every chapter. Each chapter is followed by suggested readings and references germane to the topics discussed. The experiences gleaned from running his rehabilitation program for chronic pain patients provide the reader with insights that can only be obtained through years of practice.

Dr. Vasudevan authored a superb book in 1993 aimed at those who suffer from chronic pain, and he has published extensively in the scientific literature. He has been an active participant in most of the pain-related professional societies and has served as president of many of them. He is one of a small number of physicians who espouse and implement a biopsychosocial approach to chronic pain patients, in spite of the financial difficulties that one faces when procedures are not the primary treatment strategy for chronic pain patients. The treatment program that he describes is found much more commonly in Europe than in the USA, even though it was first described and implemented in this country. Multidisciplinary pain management is more cost-effective than procedure-based care, and those countries with a rational health care system favor it over serial single-modality treatments. The biopsychosocial model is essential for the successful treatment of chronic pain patients. Hopefully, this book and the people who utilize its principles will be able to influence the funding of health care for chronic pain in the USA.

Dr. Vasudevan does a wonderful job describing multidisciplinary pain management, its components, and the strategies one can use in treating those who suffer from chronic pain. This is a resource to be treasured and deserves wide dissemination to primary care and allied practitioners.

John D. Loeser, MD
Professor, Emeritus, Neurological Surgery and Anesthesia
and Pain Medicine, University of Washington, Seattle, WA, USA
Past President of the American Pain Society
Past President of the International Association for the Study of Pain (IASP)
Washington, DC, USA

Foreword

Dr. Sridhar Vasudevan, a well-known physician who practices management of patients with chronic pain, has written a clear, concise, and understandable book on the multidisciplinary pain approach.

The book explains the "four legs" of treatment including behavioral/psychological, rehabilitation, pharmacological, and interventional approaches to chronic pain syndrome. It provides a basis for a successful philosophy behind a multidisciplinary pain approach which is an increase in function with less dependence on the health care system and more utilization of personal strategies.

The book covers successful theories behind the treatment of chronic pain including alternative techniques, common problems seen and, most compelling, the profile of patients with chronic pain syndrome. It concisely and eloquently summarizes the current theories of pain involved in the patient with chronic pain and provides the rationale for the need for multidisciplinary care.

Multidisciplinary Management of Chronic Pain: A Practical Guide for Clinicians is easy to read and understand for clinical health care personnel who evaluate and treat patients with chronic pain and will greatly help them in the understanding of the complexities and treatment of chronic pain. *This book is a "must have" reference in the office of any physician or clinician who works with patients with chronic pain.*

Martin Grabois, MD
Professor of Physical Medicine & Rehabilitation
Baylor College of Medicine, Houston, TX, USA
Medical Director
Memorial Hermann Recovery Program
Past President
American Pain Society, American Academy of Pain Medicine
American Academy of Physical Medicine & Rehabilitation
Chair Elect
American Academy of Physical Medicine & Rehabilitation, Pain Council

Acknowledgements

I would like to extend my sincere thanks to Martha Rosenberg for helping with editing of this book, providing illustrations and bringing my dreams to reality.

I am indebted to my colleagues in the field of pain medicine who have been my friends and mentors and increased the understanding and treatment of pain, helping patients everywhere.

I would like to thank the physicians who have entrusted their patients with pain to my care over four decades.

I would also like to thank the rehabilitation teams at the pain programs and hospitals where I have worked. They have helped my patients take a "different road" from that of so many chronic pain patients who are not exposed to, or not given access to, multidisciplinary pain rehabilitation programs.

I am filled with appreciation for my patients who, despite adversity, display admirable effort and tenacity in learning to their control pain and its toll on their lives.

I would like to thank my deceased parents who instilled a work ethic and spirit of volunteerism in me.

I would like to thank my sons John and Michael and my daughter-in-law Kate who have provided love over the years and my grandchildren Molly and Kate, who add meaning to my life.

I would like to thank my brother Raj who has been a friend, motivator, cheerleader and supporter for all my activities in life which has been invaluable.

I will always be grateful for my mentor John Melvin, M.D., who was my teacher and chairman of the Department of Physical Medicine & Rehabilitation at the Medical College of Wisconsin, in Milwaukee, Wisconsin, from 1974 to 1987. He encouraged my involvement in pain rehabilitation even as a resident and has remained a friend and supporter over years.

Finally, I would like to extend my sincere appreciation to Springer and my editor Ms. Janice Stern for her encouragement and patience to bring my philosophy of multidisciplinary care to treat "people with pain, and not focus on pain alone" to a wider audience.

Dr. Sridhar Vasudevan

Biography of Sridhar Vasudevan, M.D.

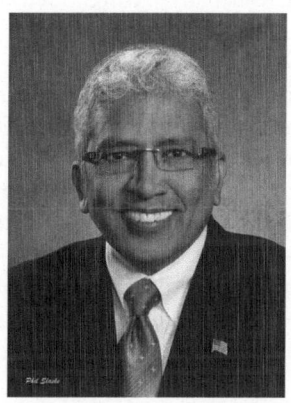

Sridhar Vasudevan graduated from the Government Medical College, in Aurangabad, India, in 1972. He completed his residency in Physical Medicine and Rehabilitation at the Medical College of Wisconsin in Milwaukee, Wisconsin, between 1974 and 1977. He is board certified in Physical Medicine and Rehabilitation as well as Pain Medicine, by the American Board of Physical Medicine and Rehabilitation. He is also board certified in Electro-diagnostic Medicine, Disability Medicine and Pain Medicine.

Vasudevan served as a full-time faculty from 1977 to 1987 in the Department. Of Physical Medicine and Rehabilitation at the **Medical College of Wisconsin** in Milwaukee, and continued as a clinical professor of PM&R in that department since 1992.

Vasudevan is **Past president** of the **Midwest Pain Society, the American Academy of Pain Medicine, the Wisconsin Society of Physical Medicine and Rehabilitation, the American College of Pain Medicine (now the American Board of Pain Medicine), and the Waukesha County Medical Society.**

He has served on the **Board of Directors** of the American Pain Society, Midwest Pain Society, Wisconsin Society of PM&R, American Academy of Pain Medicine, Waukesha County Medical Society, Sheboygan County Medical Society, the National Pain Foundation, the American Academy of Physical Medicine and Rehabilitation, Wisconsin Medical Society (WMS), the WMS Foundation and WMS Political Action Committee.

Vasudevan continues to **practice pain rehabilitation since 1977.** His current clinical practice is at the **Medical College of Wisconsin-Froedtert hospital Physical Medicine and Rehabilitation clinic**, specializing in Spine and Pain Rehabilitation, at the North Hills Health Center **in Menomonee Falls, Wisconsin.**

Vasudevan has presented several national meetings, as well as, **invited presentations at international meetings** in Israel, India, Mexico, Austria, USSR, and People's Republic of China, Germany, Aruba, Canada, Denmark, Brazil, South Africa, Australia, Turkey, Argentina and Scotland. Dr. Vasudevan continues to be active in other community volunteer activities and has served as the past president of the Father's Club of Marquette University High School, past president of the Brookfield Sunset Rotary Club, as well as the past president of Mequon-Thiensville Rotary Club and a member of the Sheboygan West Rotary Club. **He is currently an active member of the Rotary Club of Port Washington-Saukville, Wisconsin and had served on the Board of Advisors of the Feith YMCA of Port Washington-Saukville.**

He has authored several peer-reviewed articles in journals and many chapters in medical textbooks on topics of pain and disability and is an author of a book written for individuals with chronic pain and their families called **"Pain: A four letter word you can live with".**

Vasudevan was presented by the American Academy of Pain Medicine with the **Philip Lippe award** for "outstanding contributions to the social and clinical aspects of pain medicine" in February 1998. In addition he was awarded the **"Distinguished Clinician Award"** and the **"Distinguished Member Award"** by the American Academy of Physical Medicine and Rehabilitation. Dr. Vasudevan received **"The Spirit of Caring Award"** from Community Memorial Hospital/Medical Associates/advanced Health care, in Menomonee Falls in 2008.

Vasudevan is married to his supportive wife, Joyce. He is proud of his two sons. John Vasudevan, M.D (1979), who is a full time faculty member, in the department of Physical Medicine & Rehabilitation at University of Pennsylvania. His son, Michael Vasudevan (1982) works in the IT department at Marquette University, in Milwaukee, Wisconsin. He is a proud grandfather of two grand-daughters.

Contents

Chapter 1
Introduction

In this book, I will explain my personal philosophy of treating patients with chronic pain which is rooted in a multidisciplinary approach. We will also explore some popular treatments which are in wide use despite minimal evidence of their effectiveness. This book is written for clinicians—primary care physicians, physical and occupational therapists, psychologists, social workers, nurses, chiropractors and alternative healthcare providers—who see patients with chronic pain. As medical professionals, this book will help you understand the complexity of chronic pain and its treatment both which differ significantly from clinical treatment of acute pain both in practice and philosophy. It will help you guide your patients with appropriate care, education, and support to achieving and incorporating self-responsibility and self-efficacy in managing their own pain—the ultimate goal of multidisciplinary pain rehabilitation.

Academic medicine is often described as a three-legged stool balanced by one leg for teaching, patient care, and research. I like to think of pain rehabilitation as a four-legged chair with the two rear legs holding most of the weight. These strong back legs represent the behavioral/psychosocial and rehabilitation approach. The two front legs represent pharmacological and interventional/injection therapies, used as needed, and patient education/empowerment which is always needed. The seat and the rest of the chair represent the multidisciplinary team which provides a supportive environment for the individual to make the appropriate cognitive and behavioral changes and increase physical activities that are required for successful functioning despite the pain. The seat and rest of the chair, represents the patient who is surrounded with a weight-bearing system that make the chair stable (Fig. 1.1).

Another useful image is the patient with chronic pain being like a radio with two knobs. The patient is very aware of the "volume" knob and less aware of the "tuning" knob, or maybe not aware of it at all. Yet, when chronic pain is "fine-tuned," with the cafeteria of modalities offered by multidisciplinary care, the patient can tune to the right station of "relief" and improved function/control and surprisingly the *volume* of pain seems to go down as well, and certainly becomes easier to live with.

© Springer International Publishing Switzerland 2015
S. Vasudevan, *Multidisciplinary Management of Chronic Pain*,
DOI 10.1007/978-3-319-20322-5_1

Many "Supports" of Effective Pain Rehabilitation

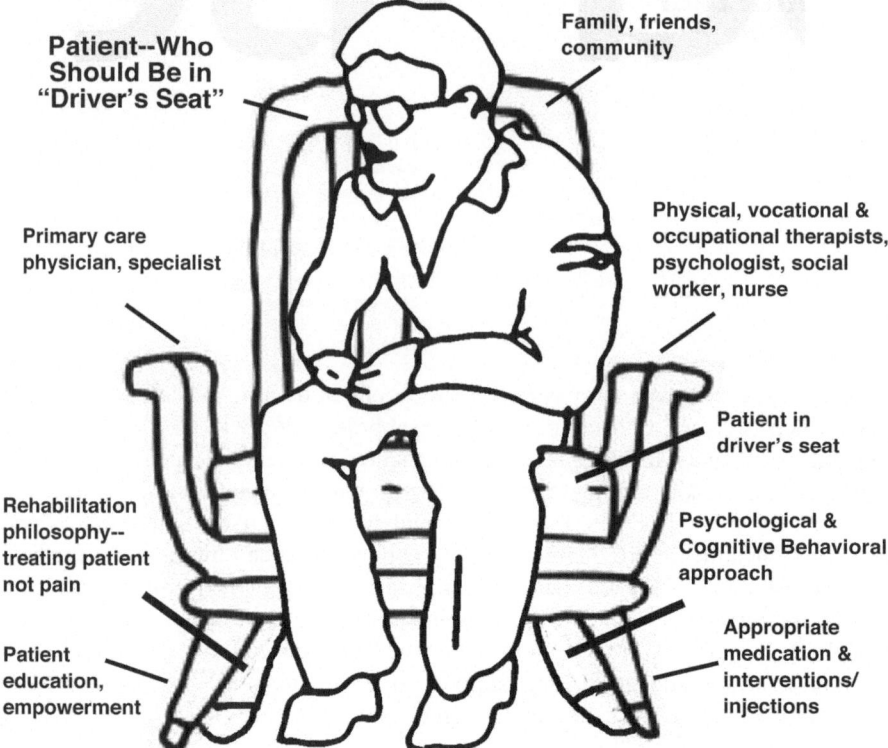

Patient--Who Should Be in "Driver's Seat"

Family, friends, community

Primary care physician, specialist

Physical, vocational & occupational therapists, psychologist, social worker, nurse

Patient in driver's seat

Rehabilitation philosophy-- treating patient not pain

Psychological & Cognitive Behavioral approach

Patient education, empowerment

Appropriate medication & interventions/ injections

Fig. 1.1 Many "supports" of effective pain rehabilitation

The result is an increase in function with less dependence on the healthcare system and disability systems (Fig. 1.2).

Many of the patients we see have had pain for months or years and repeatedly sought surgery, opioids and intervention treatments without effectiveness or positive outcomes. As more and more medical professionals have thrown up their hands at their patients with chronic pain conditions, these patients have lost hope and some have become despondent, depressed, and/or desperate.

In my years of practice I have had the opportunity to see and participate in the rehabilitation of more than 10,000 patients with chronic or persistent pain. Most of these patients have not responded to treatment with medications, surgery, anesthesia interventions, prescription drugs (mainly opioids/narcotics), chiropractic care and complementary and alternative medicine (CAM) techniques.

Most of these individuals have become dependent on medications even though they also usually say the medication is not helpful. They have become dependent on the healthcare system and continue to seek evaluations and treatment, hoping for the "fix" which only lead to despondency and failure. Constant pain has become a com-

How Chronic Pain Is Like a Radio

Most patients are more aware of the "volume" knob on their pain than the "tuning" knob. Yet, when pain is "fine-tuned" with multidisciplinary modalities, patients can tune to the right "station" of relief and improved function and control and surprisingly the volume of pain seems to go down.

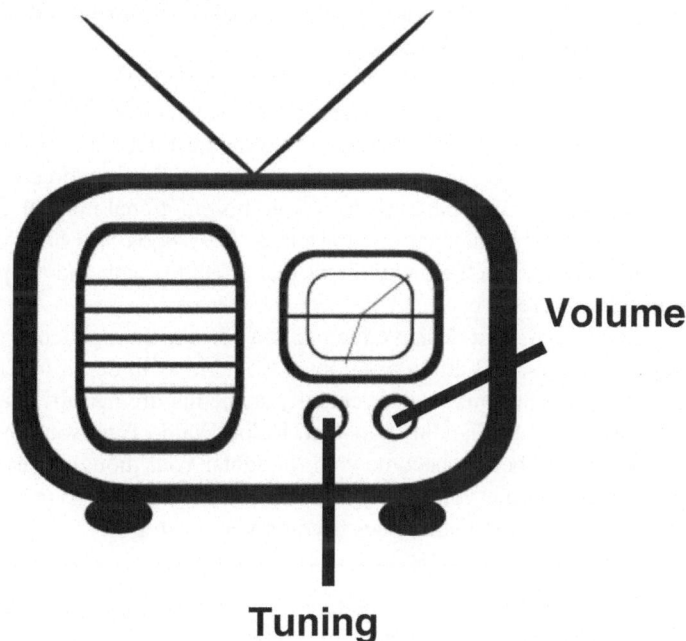

Fig. 1.2 How chronic pain is like a radio

pelling force in their lives, incapacitating them from the roles they had once performed as workers, spouses, parents, and homemakers. Many have become full-time patients who think of themselves as disabled individuals. *Yet these patients make astounding improvements when given a different "road" than the one they have been on: multidisciplinary pain rehabilitation.*

Treating the Person Not the "Pain"

Chronic pain is a growing problem for patients and society as a whole. The many new books, scientific journals and government/medical task forces addressing chronic pain reveal the increase in growth and numbers of persons with chronic pain which frustrates patients and medical professionals alike. Despite medications, surgery and physical and anesthesiology interventions, the number of adults reporting chronic pain is increasing, as we explore in Chaps. 1 and 4. In this book, you will see how the very way chronic pain is currently regarded, as a purely biomedical experience to be treated with single, unimodal therapies instead of multidisciplinary, is behind the poor outcomes. There are only six ways to treat chronic pain, which we explore in Chap. 6: pharmaceuticals, interventions/injections done by anesthesiologists and other pain specialists, surgery, physical therapy modalities psychological approaches, and multidisciplinary rehabilitation. Significantly, a multidisciplinary approach is the only treatment that *encompasses all of the other four modalities* which explains its effectiveness.

There is no question that social, psychological, and environmental factors exert profound effects on chronic pain. These factors, which are often out of your patient's awareness and control, are the reason unimodal interventions often fail and why multidisciplinary care is often remarkably successful: it addresses the vast web of factors that influence a patient's pain from his emotional makeup and family life to his vocational and financial circumstances. This book will help you acquaint you and your patient with the many forces that affect his pain and adopt a new, positive attitude toward recovery.

Arguably, the most decisive factors in a chronic pain patient's prognosis are his thoughts, beliefs, and attitudes—topics we address in depth in Chaps. 2, 3 and 4. The way a patient thinks will eventually shape his life narrative says the following quote, attributed to Gandhi, Lao Tzu, Ralph Waldo Emerson, and even Margaret Thatcher: "Your beliefs become your thoughts; Your thoughts become your words; Your words become your actions; Your actions become your habits; Your habits become your values; Your values become your destiny."

> "Your beliefs become your thoughts; Your thoughts become your words; Your words become your actions; Your actions become your habits; Your habits become your values; Your values become your destiny"

Most pain patients believe four "truisms" (see Table 1.1) about their pain which are *not true at all* for chronic pain (though they may be true for acute pain). As we treat, educate, and support patients in self-efficacy and self-management, we help them turn these misconceptions into a realistic view of their pain condition and how best to live with it.

Table 1.1 Patients' chronic pain misconceptions/beliefs and realities

Misconceptions/beliefs	Realties
Pain indicates something is wrong	Pain is not always from a problem that can be diagnosed and treated
Pain always has a cause that can be discovered	Even when the cause of pain is known, X-rays and blood tests may not reveal it
Pain indicates a condition which can be cured	Even when a cause of the pain is known, a permanent "cure" often doesn't exist
After pain is resolved, a patient should be able to return to normal functioning	Although pain may never go away and affect certain functions, patients can gain control over their pain and improve overall functional levels

In this book, you will see that the phenomenon of chronic pain is so complex, scientists do not fully understand it and clinicians cannot "cure" it. While there are many plausible theories of etiology, which we explore in detail in Chap. 3, much chronic pain is not explained by the major theories.

You will also see that the treatments for acute and chronic pain differ and, in some cases, are opposites. While rest and passivity are often the key features of the treatment of acute pain, chronic pain management calls for activity and exercise. Notably, the medications given for acute pain may make chronic pain worse. Medications which will help chronic pain patients are discussed in Chap. 6.

Experiencing Pain Personally

On a personal level, I have experienced the disabling results of chronic pain which gives me great empathy for pain patients. Starting in my early teenage years, I experienced headaches which began intermittently but became a daily problem. Evaluations revealed that I required glasses and corrective lenses were prescribed. This initially helped some aspects of the headaches but the severe throbbing continued over the years and to this day. This allows me to relate to my patients' frustration when treatments don't work or work well.

After visiting a round of physicians, my headaches were diagnosed as migraines but they proved refractory to all the medications I was prescribed. While I was in medical school and later, in my residency, the migraines persisted. In my teens and early 20s, while going to medical school, I was also involved in several motorcycle accidents and other falls. This resulted in several fractures, as well as many softtissue injuries. I was left with chronic softtissue pains, which were unexplained. Currently, these are best understood as regional myofascial pain syndromes, predominantly involving the cervical and scapular muscles, and, to a lesser degree, the lumbar paraspinal muscles. These daily aches and pains have continued till today.

Surrounded by my medical colleagues I received ample advice about medications to try but still none worked to relieve the persistent pain of my headaches. Like the patients I continued to seek a "better" diagnosis and treatment because the pain continued!

Finally after a brain scan revealed no physical cause of the pain and no significant medical problems, I was given the diagnosis of a "mixed headache disorder with muscle tension type headaches and migraine." Luckily for me, a physician who thought "out of the box," suggested that I try treatments other than medication. He set me on a path of stretching exercises, stress relieving exercises, and diversion techniques that works to relieve my headaches to this day. These are many of the same treatment modalities offered in this book.

By recognizing that stress provoked my headaches, using nonnarcotic medications and applying manual physical therapy, stretching, regular exercises, and the cognitive behavioral and relaxation techniques in Chap. 4 of this book, I was able to pursue my dream of a career in rehabilitation medicine. I control my chronic pain with stretching, physical modalities such as heat and home massage and rare over-the-counter NSAIDs and muscle relaxants which is the same advice I give patients. Blending these different treatments has enabled me to fulfill my role as a physician, as a father, and husband. I have been able to help my patients and students by teaching the concepts of pain management I have been privileged to learn and practice with my own pain conditions. Remembering with gratitude, how a physician placed me on a better road to pain management, I have tried to similarly guide my patients in these techniques and, with this book, other medical professionals.

Toward a New Attitude Toward Chronic Pain

Pain has existed since prehistoric times and, as we note in Chap. 3 which explores predominant pain theories, still presents many ambiguities. We do not know why pain can be absent, as when a soldier does not notice a grave injury in battle or why it can be present with no apparent physical cause.

In the last decades there have been many advancements in the understanding and treatment of chronic pain. Yet, as we will explore in Chap. 5, only about 20 % of contemporary pain treatments, which tend to be unimodal rather than multidisciplinary, are evidence-based. Many treatments prove ineffective, need to be repeated or need additional treatments added to them.

Like few other medical fields, problem solving is at the basis of chronic pain management—for both medical professionals and patients seeking to surmount their pain. The patients who improve the most are those who accept the fact that there are no "quick fixes" or cures in pain management.

When I sense a patient is impatient and wants instant results, I remind him of all the famous people in history who only found success after years of failures and disappointments. It took Darwin his entire lifetime to develop his theory of evolution. Randolph Hearst, the publishing icon, recounts how the first article he wrote was rejected by 36 different publications. It is said that Beethoven wrote and rewrote his first major symphony 20 times and that Thomas Edison tried his first light bulb 20,000 times before it worked. Abraham Lincoln failed at many of his efforts initially, but persisted in his dreams to become one of the greatest American Presidents of all times. Citing these famous people, I try to help patients find new sources of motivation, determination and willingness in their path to manage chronic pain.

Whether or not the pain patient realizes it, he has a choice in the attitude he decides to adopt. Throughout this book, I have used the term "he" for brevity but obviously patients are of both genders. He can continue on his road of frustrations and disappointment, feeling increasingly hopeless that his pain will ever lessen. He can think of himself as a victim of pain and treatments that don't work and dwell on his pain. Or, the patient can decide to move forward and, no longer "do the same thing but expect different results," as insanity is sometimes described. He can decide he is "sick and tired of being sick and tired." He can become open minded to a new path of pain management.

Pain is an intensely personal experience. Just as no one can understand our patient's pain, no one can *manage* it but the patient, because he lives with it on a day-to-day basis. Yet, because it is a crisis, chronic pain can also present new opportunities in our patients' lives. Unable to stay on a path of pain management that is frustrating and disappointing, a patient is forced to change in a medical "sink or swim" situation. Being forced to change presents opportunities for patients to reevaluate and refocus their lives, tapping into new sources of energy and making new commitments. As Lao Tzu, the famous philosopher and poet notes: "If you do not change direction you may end up where you were heading."

To some of the patients with chronic pain, where they are heading is the road that leads to drug dependence, disuse, depression, and disability from most activities. However, clinicians working with the multidisciplinary model are also pleased to see one patient who decides to go back to college, another who renews a commitment to a marriage that did not appear viable and another patient who decides to pursue a new career path he never thought possible. I often wonder if the patients would have taken these exciting and life-affirming steps without their pain crisis.

One of the rewards of working in rehabilitation is I see patients who come into my office in wheelchairs and grimacing in pain move with new ease in a relatively short period of time from accepting a multidisciplinary treatment approach and learning new methods of coping. I remember a particular elderly woman who first came to my office in a wheelchair. Disabled by osteoarthritis, she never expected to walk again. But just weeks later, after working with our multidisciplinary pain team, she was bouncing down the halls in tennis shoes and a sweat suit. What was the variable? She began to dream again, to give up her pessimism and enlarge her realm of possibility. Of course a dramatic recovery like hers is not always possible—but the fact of such transformations happen, should give both patients and the clinicians inspiration and hope.

In many ways, this book is about just such dreams—the dreams of your patients. They dream of being whole again, living their lives to the fullest and being the best that they can be despite their discouraging battles with chronic pain. If the patient is committed, he can know the options available, know himself better and achieve control over his pain. Again to quote, Lao Tzu, "Knowing others is intelligence; knowing yourself is wisdom." He also noted that, "To hold you must first open your hand and let go" and "The journey of a thousand miles begins with the first step."

You as a medical professional can help patients by introducing them to a new path and the steps to managing their pain. By making them a partner in the journey, you will see a transformation in the patient contained in this proverb. "I hear and I forget; I see and I remember; I do and I understand."

I hear and I forget

I see and I remember

I do and I understand

Looking Ahead

As this book goes to press, a federal advisory group has rolled out a National Pain Strategy (NPS) for public comment which corroborates the precepts in this book, from the value of multidisciplinary and biopsychosocial approaches to pain to the importance of patient self-management.

A unified effort of the FDA, National Institutes of Health (NIH), Centers for Disease Control and Prevention (CDC), Departments of Defense and Veterans Affairs and the Agency for Healthcare Research and Quality, the advisory group, called the Interagency Pain Research Coordinating Committee (IPRCC), seeks to enact the Affordable Care Act goal of increasing "the recognition of pain as a significant public health problem" (IPRCC 2015).

Among the objectives in the NPS's vision statement are better education for pain patients about "effective approaches for self-care and pain self-management programs that would help them prevent, cope with, and reduce pain and its disability," a better patient understanding of the "benefits and risks of pain management options," greater "self-care interventions" for patients and greater use of coordinated, multidisciplinary care by clinicians.

Included in the NPS vision strategy is the goal of clinicians taking "active prevention measures to prevent the progression of acute to chronic pain and its associated disabilities."

As expressed in many sections of this book, the NPS report indicts excessive use of non evidence-based treatments in the worsening of our national pain problem, including the irresponsible use of opioids. It notes "the lack of financial incentives for healthcare providers to promote multimodal and interdisciplinary approaches to pain management," Robert Kerns, Ph.D., of Yale and the Connecticut, VA, who chaired one of the report panels, told MedPage Today (2015).

"Because commonly used single-modality treatments often fail as first-line therapies for chronic pain, attention among leaders in the field has shifted to improving pain assessment and delivery of integrated, multimodal, interdisciplinary care that is effective and safe," says the report. As such, NPS objectives include promoting "coordinated care across the continuum of pain in order to conform to the biopsychosocial model and provide value, as defined by outcomes of care," "incentiviz[ing] high-quality, coordinated pain care through an integrated biopsychosocial approach that is cost-effective" and a "national educational campaign encouraging safe medication use, especially opioid use, among patients with pain."

The NPS recommendations are good news for pain patients and the clinicians who see them. They echo what I have learned in my decades of practice and share in this book. However, there are two hurdles to overcome before patients will begin benefiting from these important government objectives. One is the long duration of time that will no doubt be necessary before strategy is implemented and the other is the ever-present likelihood of special medical interest groups chipping away at the recommendations to keep ineffective but lucrative pain therapies first-line. Readers of this book will no doubt share with me the hope that reimbursement models will be firmly put in place to support treating chronic pain patients with what we know is the optimal treatment: multidisciplinary pain rehabilitation programs.

References

Fiore, K. (2015, April 4). Is pain a public health crisis?—Federal advisory group wants to frame chronic pain as public health problem. *MedPage Today*.

Interagency Pain Research Coordinating Committee. (2015). *A comprehensive population health-level strategy for pain: national pain strategy*. Washington, DC: Interagency Pain Research Coordinating Committee.

Lao Tzu. Quotation. Brainy Quote. Retrieved from http://www.brainyquote.com/quotes/quotes/l/laotzu121075.html

Mahatma Gandhi. Quotation. The Quotations Page. Retrieved from http://www.quotationspage.com/quote/36464.html

Chapter 2
The Problem of Chronic Pain

Demystifying Pain for Your Patients

Anyone who works in the medical field knows the toll chronic pain exerts on patients firsthand. Often when you first see a pain patient, he already has a long list of providers he has seen and treatments that have failed. (In this book we are using "he" when referring to patients for brevity, while obviously patients are both genders.) He often brings to the visit not only a long and discouraging narrative but an increasingly despondent emotional state. He may feel his pain is not being taken seriously, that no one is "listening" to him and that no one understands him. He may be nurturing resentments against employers and insurance companies if his pain resulted from an accident or injury and be harboring strong feelings of self-pity.

Many chronic pain patients have stopped working and limited their life activities out of fear that their pain will worsen—a fear which ironically makes pain worse as we will explore in subsequent chapters. They have become isolated and irritable and their family relations have become strained. Their eating and sleeping behaviors have often become dysfunctional and they may be catapulting toward depression, if they are not already clinically depressed. They have likely adopted verbal or nonverbal pain "behaviors" like sighing and grimacing which perpetuate the pain portrayal to others—and themselves. When you see such a patient, you often inherit the disappointing pain outcomes he has already endured and his increasing feelings of pessimism and skepticism.

Both patients and physicians are at a knowledge disadvantage when it comes to treating chronic pain. Pain patients often pursue a "cure" or quick "fix"/treatment for years, stubbornly resistant to changing their perspective or expectations. Ironically, it is only when they accept that a pure "cure" is not feasible and learn more about the complexities of pain that improvements will be seen.

Physicians, for their part, receive only a few hours of training about chronic pain and less than 4 % of US medical schools require a course in pain (Ochoa 2012).

© Springer International Publishing Switzerland 2015
S. Vasudevan, *Multidisciplinary Management of Chronic Pain*,
DOI 10.1007/978-3-319-20322-5_2

Table 2.1 Chronic pain facts

1.   Chronic pain is seldom "cured" but can be managed effectively
2.   Unlike nociceptive pain, chronic pain serves no clear biological "purpose"
3.   We do not fully understand the cause of all patients with chronic pain
4.   The existence of pain cannot be proved
5.   There is little correlation between pain and disability or impairment
6.   Chronic pain often confounds unimodal, symptomatic treatment
7.   A multidisciplinary treatment approach to pain is frequently most effective

Consequently, many physicians neither fully understand pain nor enjoy treating chronic pain patients as opposed to acute pain patients who improve predictably. Certainly, we, as medical professionals, are trained to not be comfortable admitting we "don't know" the etiology of condition or that we have limited ability to treat it. We are frustrated when we can't help patients in the way we wish to help.

The truth is that medical science neither offers a full explanation of the development of chronic nonmalignant pain or how to eliminate it as we see in Table 2.1. We do not recognize any biological purpose it serves and we cannot identify clear correlations between pain and disability, despite patients who clearly appear to be in pain and are often not working or leading functional lives.

Nor is chronic pain the public health priority it should be. Over 100 million Americans experience chronic pain and its treatment costs the US$635 billion a year—compared with heart disease ($309 billion), cancer ($243 billion), and diabetes ($188 billion) (Institute of Medicine 2011). Chronic pain represents $11.6–$12.7 billion a year in lost work days in the United States with many workers not returning at all. Yet, of the 27 institutes in the National Institutes of Health (NIH) not one is dedicated to pain.

Two Different Roads to Pain Management

We have all heard that there are many "different roads to Rome." Similarly, there are many roads to managing pain and most pain patients you will see are on the undesirable "road" of narcotics, injections, surgery, rest from activity, disability, anticipatory fear, activity avoidance, and excessive focusing on their pain, often with the encouragement of their family. When people when they think of a "road less traveled" many remember the beautiful poem by Robert Frost, called The Road Not Taken on the topic, and pictured in Fig. 2.1 (2002)

Acknowledge that you believe the patient's pain is real
Ascertain the patient's previous treatments, experience and "pain story"
Help the patient see his pain is affected by body, mind and social/situational factors
Connect the patient with others on a multidisciplinary team who can help
Convey that a new "path" exists for pain management that requires a new attitude
Enlist the patient as a member and mutual decision maker on the treatment team

Fig. 2.1 Getting started with a pain patient

The Road Not Taken
By Robert Frost

Two roads diverged in a yellow wood,
And sorry I could not travel both
And be one traveler, long I stood
And looked down one as far as I could
To where it bent in the undergrowth;

Then took the other, as just as fair,
And having perhaps the better claim,
Because it was grassy and wanted wear;
Though as for that the passing there
Had worn them really about the same,

And both that morning equally lay
In leaves no step had trodden black.
Oh, I kept the first for another day!
Yet knowing how way leads on to way,
I doubted if I should ever come back.

I shall be telling this with a sigh
Somewhere ages and ages hence:
Two roads diverged in a wood, and I—
I took the one less traveled by,
And that has made all the difference. (2002 Owl)

But too often this "road" is characterized by uncoordinated medical care and unimodal treatments that are not evidence-based as we see in Table 2.2. In fact, despite today's arsenal of popular new pain treatments, the incidence of adults who report chronic pain has grown from 50 million a few decades ago to 100 million (Wells-Federman 1999; American Academy of Pain Medicine 2011). Clearly, this road is not working.

The multidisciplinary pain rehabilitation road is less traveled but infinitely more effective. It involves elimination of narcotics (which are seldom useful in chronic pain), identification of appropriate medication(s), addressing the patient's psychological, social and emotional issues and educating the patient about pain and pain management. Rather than the "cure" for chronic pain which patients have sought in surgery or medications, the multidisciplinary road offers them a "cafeteria" of treat-

Table 2.2 Signs of ineffective pain management

1. Narcotic use without increased function
2. Repeated injections
3. Repeated surgery
4. Rest instead of activity
5. Disability
6. Fear of pain and activities
7. Focus on pain
8. Worsening mood—depression, anger, helplessness, hopelessness

ments from different disciplines. These include different medications such as anti-depressants and antiseizure drugs, education and empowerment, physical therapy such as stretching, self-mobilization and aerobic exercises, strengthening and endurance building and Transcutaneous Electrical Nerve Stimulation (TENS) or cognitive and behavioral techniques like altering thought patterns, distraction and mental imagery.

> The goal of multidisciplinary pain rehabilitation is to induce in the patient a sense of self-efficacy and self-responsibility as a partner in his own pain management

The goal of multidisciplinary pain rehabilitation is to induce in the patient a sense of self-efficacy and self-responsibility as a partner in his own pain management. This happens as the patient is taught how to increase activities at work or home without fear or strain and how to achieve a new perspective of his pain and life through working with a psychologist, when needed. As patients are empowered by members of the multidisciplinary team, they learn self-management and are able to control their pain instead of having it "control" them. Often there is an "aha" moment or a Gestalt in which the patient realizes that recovery is up to him and he participates in the treatment in a new way.

Of course treating chronic pain with a multidisciplinary rather than traditional approach is not without controversy. There are also intense philosophical conflicts regarding the treatment of chronic pain which we will explore in this book.

Chronic Pain Is a Biopsychosocial Process

Many trace the multidisciplinary team concept to Tacoma General Hospital where John Bonica, an anesthesiologist, and his colleagues recognized that chronic pain patients needed more than a physician to improve their function in the 1940s. Dr. Bonica recruited a group consisting of John D. Loeser, M.D., a neurosurgeon,

Table 2.3 Distinguishing features of multidisciplinary approach

Conventional	Multidisciplinary
Pain relief	Functional improvement
Peripheral treatment	Central and peripheral treatment
Opioid drugs	Minimal or no opioid drugs
Surgery	Minimally invasive procedures
Unimodal treatment	Multimodal rehabilitation
Patient care	Patient responsibility
Passive care	Active participation
Expensive, non-EMB care	Cost-effective, EBM care

Wilbert Fordyce, Ph.D., a psychologist, a physiatrist, and physical and occupational therapists and sought to develop a biopsychosocial model of pain management (IASP 2012). Interestingly, the new approach focused on improving function as opposed to eliminating pain.

Treating a patient with a team of professionals including the patient himself and ideally the patient's family has two salutary results. It produces *coordinated* care in which the "left hand knows what the right hand is doing" (a feature that is seriously lacking in our healthcare system) and it enfolds the patient in decision-making process. The key differences between conventional and multidisciplinary treatment are shown in Table 2.3.

Let the Patient Drive the Bus

"A treatment that is simply handed to a patient without his or her input....is less likely to work or be adhered to," says Scott M. Fishman, M.D. one of the nation's leading pain experts and author of several pain texts (Fishman 2012a, b, p. 67). "Patients are best served by being put in the role of chief executive officer of their treatment regimens," he writes.

When first instituted, pain programs with multidisciplinary teams flourished in the United States. Teams could include physical and occupational therapists, exercise physiologists, rehabilitation nurses, social workers, vocational therapists, therapeutic recreation therapists, ergonomics specialists, dieticians, pharmacists, and even members of the clergy. The multidisciplinary pain programs, also called interdisciplinary programs, were a good example of holistic medicine—treating the person not just the symptoms. They exemplified a biopsychosocial approach to health in which the body and the brain are acknowledged to be interconnected and work together. But sadly, due to a shifting healthcare reimbursement environment, multidisciplinary pain programs are disappearing in United States even as their popularity grows in the rest of the world.

John D. Loeser, M.D. one of Dr. Bonica's original team members and considered a leader in the multidisciplinary pain approach today in the United States, has

Table 2.4   Chronic pain precepts in multidisciplinary care

1.   Chronic pain must be viewed as a mind/body, and biopsychosocial and cultural occurrence
2.   Chronic pain cannot be treated like acute pain with passive rest and modalities
3.   Patients must understand what "hurts" them does not necessarily "harm" them
4.   Patients who become active participants in their treatments generally improve

lamented how multidisciplinary rehabilitation in the United States is disappearing due to overreliance on narcotic pain killers. "This often occurs with little or no attempt to assess patients' real needs, as if chronic pain were a purely medical problem and psychological and social factors of no account," he said in the International Association for the Study of Pain's magazine *Insight* (2013). Four key precepts of multidisciplinary treatment are seen in Table 2.4.

The Pain Management Pendulum Has Swung Back

It is noteworthy that before the idea of a multidisciplinary team developed, chronic pain was regarded as a purely medical problem—and the pendulum has swung back. Then and now, treatment is too often focused on masking the pain with anti-anxiety drugs, narcotic pain drugs, injections and surgery without probing emotional and cultural factors—literally "treating the pain and not the patient." Treatments like spinal fusions and disk surgery, spinal cord stimulators, steroid and painkiller injections, nerve ablation, and of course long-term prescription of narcotics have become the norm in pain care, especially in the United States. At the same time, the incidence of adults who report chronic pain has doubled. Clearly, the newer methods are not working.

It should be no surprise that changes in the way health care is delivered and reimbursed are at the heart of these changes. Chronic pain treatment in the United States is increasingly "dictated by what insurance providers will pay for rather than by individual patient needs," and, at best, such treatment is "inappropriate, and at worst is dangerous," maintains Dr. Loeser, who is Professor Emeritus, of neurological surgery, anesthesiology and pain medicine at the University of Washington. "Health professionals, not insurance providers or managers and politicians, must once again be in charge of medical planning and decision making."

Lynn Webster, M.D., former president of the American Academy of Pain Medicine (AAPM) agrees. "All payers should offer a comprehensive, interdisciplinary pain program to patients who have disabling pain," wrote Dr. Webster in an article titled, "We Have an Epidemic on Our Hands and the Status Quo Is Failing Us" in *Pain Medicine News* (Webster 2013) . "In addition, all payers should make available cognitive behavioral therapy to people with chronic pain. At minimum, these benefits should be similar to the 2008 federal law mandating parity for mental health treatment." I strongly agree with his Dr. Webster's statement.

In addition to inappropriate and uncoordinated care, current pain care also emphasizes short-term savings at the price of long-term results, writes Barry Meier, a *New York Times* reporter. "In the short run, treating a patient with an opioid like OxyContin, which costs about $6000 a year, is less expensive than putting a patient through a pain-treatment program that emphasizes physical therapy and behavior modification," but over time multidisciplinary programs "might yield far lower costs," he observes.

An average worker compensation claim without opioids, for example, is $13,000 but leaps to $39,000 when short-acting opioids are added and $117,000 when long-acting opioids are added (Meier 2013). According to a study by the California Workers' Compensation Institute, workers who received high opioid doses stayed out of work *three times longer* than those who took lower doses, "What we see is an association between the greater use of opioids and delayed recovery from workplace injuries," explained Alex Swedlow, head of research at the Institute (Meier 2013).

A 2008 study in the journal *Spine* found people kept on opioids for more than 7 days during the first 6 weeks after an injury were more than *twice as likely to be disabled and out of work a year later* (Fauber and Gabler 2012). A study of 300,000 Workers' Compensation claims by the Workers Compensation Research Institute found pain and day-to-day function do not improve in workers when they stay on opioids (Fauber 2012).

Multidisciplinary pain rehabilitation, on the other hand, is effective for pain patients and cost-effective for providers according to medical literature. The "multidisciplinary treatment ameliorates pain, functional restoration, and quality of life with medium to high-effect sizes even for patients with a long history of chronic back pain," says a paper in the *Journal of Clinical Rheumatology* (Moradi et al. 2012). "Results demonstrate that participation in a [multidisciplinary] chronic pain program is an effective intervention for selected patients with refractory pain," echoes a study in *Pain Physician* (McAllister et al. 2005). "Primary care-based treatment of chronic pain by interdisciplinary teams (including behavioral specialists, nurse case managers, physical therapists, and pharmacists) is one of the most effective approaches for improving outcomes and managing costs," concluded an article in *Translational Behavioral Medicine* (Debar et al. 2012).

In Denmark, implementation of clinics with multidisciplinary teams cut the rate of lumbar disk surgery in half in just 4 years. (Rasmussen et al. 2005). Before the team-based clinics, patients with low back pain (LBP) were "referred unsystematically to various diagnostic methods," write the authors in a 2005 article in *Spine* and there was a "high degree of uncertainty about both diagnosis and prognosis." After the multidisciplinary nonsurgical spine clinics were in operation, patients benefited from a faster and more "competent evaluation," an education program geared to general physicians that stressed "the benefits of a more conservative approach" and a "local media campaign stressing the concept of 'watchful waiting.'"

Table 2.5 The six ways of treating chronic pain

1. Pharmaceutical (painkillers, antidepressants, antiseizure drugs)
2. Interventional (injections, nerve blocks, neuromodulation)
3. Surgically (to eliminate or stabilize)
4. Physical modalities (physical therapy, acupuncture, etc.)
5. Psychological (cognitive behavioral, relaxation therapy)
6. A combination of all the above

Remembering the Words of Hippocrates

There are six ways to treat chronic pain as seen in Table 2.5. The first three—drugs, interventions (injections, nerve block, spinal cord stimulators, and Intrathecal drug delivery systems) and surgery—are seen together. But they are seldom blended with psychological treatment and a multidisciplinary approach. It is ironic and unfortunate that when most patients think of pain treatments, they think of an individual modality like injections and seldom about a combination of therapies to get the right "blend."

Worse, both patients and physicians have embraced expensive and high-tech pain treatments which are not evidence-based, as we will address in subsequent chapters.

Almost from the first day of medical school, physicians learn two sayings from the father of medicine, Hippocrates: "First, do no harm" and "comfort always." Clearly medical professionals need to ensure that "bad things" that may need surgery or acute treatment are addressed promptly while allowing "nature" to take care of self-limiting conditions. Those conditions like most muscle strains and sprains, and minor fractures will heal with appropriate time and medications, support, or heat or cold to make the patient more comfortable in his recovery process.

The Dangers of the "X-ray Diagnosis"

Unfortunately, the phenomenon of readily accessible X-rays and other imaging technologies has increased our capacity to, unwittingly, "do harm" through dispensing poor prognoses, diagnostic labels, and misattributing pain symptoms. In almost all cases, abnormalities and age-related changes shown on X-rays and MRIs are not the source of the patient's pain. Yet, 75 % of patients over 50 are told they have "thinning of the discs" and 60 % of patients as young as 30 are told they have "arthritis" on the basis of X-rays and MRI scans This misattribution can be disturbing and harmful to patients and lead to treatments they may not need.

The truth is the so-called "arthritis," disk "thinning," "degenerative disk disease" and a "bulging" disk are usually as predictable and expected as graying hair; a natural part of aging and not a medical problem. We certainly don't call gray hair "follicular depigmentation syndrome" and treat it aggressively.

These diagnoses can be terrifying and take on the power of urban legends writes David Hanscom, M.D. in *Back in Control* (2012). "I recall one sixty-year-old gentleman I saw many years ago who'd been experiencing back pain for about eight weeks. He was terrified because he'd been told he had degenerated disks. He feared paralysis and loss of function," writes Dr. Hanscom. "I explained to him in detail that his spine was *completely* normal for his age. As I pointed out earlier….there is no correlation between degenerated disks and back pain."

Surgeons tend to believe that if a structural "pain generator" can be identified, the "pain will resolve," writes Dr. Hanscom. While on the surface this seems plausible, in point of fact "physicians can make an exact diagnosis of the source of lower back pain only about fifteen percent of the time (2012, p. 3)."

Often what is identified on the scan as the pain generator is not the source of the patient's pain—and would not have caused pain if its presence weren't known. In low back pain (LBP) sufferers, 90 % of X-rays or MRIs show no specific structural abnormalities, nor do nerve tests or neurological examinations pinpoint the pain source. Moreover, from 40 to 60 % of asymptomatic patients show abnormal X-ray changes when imagery is done for other reasons.

When interpreting an X-ray, medical professionals should first assure a patient that there is no evidence of fracture, tumors/cancer or progressive instability before discussing any middle-age-related arthritis which is revealed (and is likely not the source of the patient's pain). Many current treatment guidelines strongly suggest refraining from X-rays for at least for 4–6 weeks after a episode of acute back or neck pain for this reason—to avoid conferring an upsetting "X-ray diagnosis" upon a patient that may not have relevance to a pain condition.

Early or unnecessary imaging has been linked to unwanted outcomes in the medical literature. "Excessive use of spine imaging may contribute to the problem" of unneeded or excessive surgery noted a paper in the *European Spine Journal*, "along with unrealistic patient expectations, a desire to validate disability claims, or wishful thinking on the part of both doctors and patients." "Early MRI may lead to greater subsequent interventions, potentially poorer outcomes, and increased health care expenditures," echoes a paper in the journal *Spine*. Sadly, there may be "financial incentives for hospitals, surgeons, and device manufacturers" to overuse MRIs observes the *European Spine Journal* and Reuters has found that MRIs are ordered more frequently when health care providers have a financial stake in the imaging center or the equipment used.

Nortin Hadler, M.D., Attending Rheumatologist at the University of North Carolina Hospitals and author of *Worried Sick* (2008) and *Stabbed in the Back*: *Confronting Back Pain in an Overtreated Society* (2009), writes that "billions of dollars are spent annually in the pointless exercise" of unnecessary diagnostic scans (2009).

"Who among us can look at an image of our own spine and not feel disquiet as we come to realize how many disks have degenerated, how many facet joints have spurs, how peculiar is the alignment? What has gone wrong? What will happen to me? What did I do? What should I avoid?" he writes. "Given the common horror of disease, these queries and the accompanying angst are predictable. We all need to be disabused."

Jerome Groopman, M.D., Professor of Medicine at Harvard Medical School, Chief of Experimental Medicine at Beth Israel Deaconess Medical Center and author of *How Doctors Think* (2007) voices similar reservations, especially about the ability of X-rays to "generate false positives" and for "normal structures" to be labeled "abnormal." Dr. Groopman quotes E. James Potchen, M.D., of Michigan State University who has studied X-ray reliability warning medical professionals that, "if you look at a film too long, you increase the risk of hurting the patient (p. 180).

Acute Versus Chronic Pain Treatment

We medical professionals excel at treating acute conditions like a broken leg, chest pain, appendicitis or infection that have clear explanations and protocols.

Chronic conditions, on the other hand, like diabetes mellitus, hypertension, asthma, Parkinson's disease, migraine headaches and, of course, chronic pain usually have no specific "cause" or "cure" and do not resolve predictably like acute conditions do, with time and treatment. Even when chronic conditions *do* have a clear "cause" such as post-herpetic neuralgia from shingles, there is still seldom a "cure" we can offer patients. While we know the nerves in these patients have been "rewired" due to chemical, physiological and even anatomical changes which result in the burning and shooting pains they report, we can generally manage these overactive nerves rather than "cure" them.

Over 40 years ago, the medical field recognized that managing chronic pain is not only different from managing acute pain, the treatment for the two kinds of pain are polar opposites. While rest is recommended for acute pain, chronic pain requires activity. While narcotics and passive therapies like injections, multiple surgeries, chiropractic and opioid medications are appropriate for acute pain, they are not appropriate in chronic pain. In some select chronic pain patients, narcotic pain medications may improve quality of life, when used according to established guidelines established by the Federation of State Medical Boards but usually, when used long-term, they worsen pain and can lead to drug dependence and addiction (Fishman 2012a, b, 2014).

There is another difference in the treatment of acute versus chronic pain and it is a philosophical one. In acute pain, the patient is treated with passive modalities that do not require his participation—"nature" does the healing. In chronic pain management, on the other hand, the patient *has* to become an active participant in the care for improvement to result. When a chronic pain patient is *not* an active participant

Table 2.6 Many chronic pain patients exhibit theses "Ds"

Dramatic verbal/nonverbal pain behaviors
Disability out of proportion to medical findings
Disuse of an extremity
Dysfunction of the body part and social roles
Depression—anger, hopelessness
Deconditioning
Discouragement
Despair
Drug abuse—especially with opioids/narcotics
Dependency on family; healthcare system

in his care, he usually develops a condition characterized by many Ds: Dramatic pain behaviors, Disability conviction, Disuse of an extremity, Dysfunction, Depression, Deconditioning, Discouragement, Despair, Drug abuse, and, above all, Dependency on family and the healthcare system. Most of us have seen the "Ds" firsthand in our offices, as shown in Table 2.6.

One of the best things you can do for your chronic patient is to clearly explain the difference between "hurt" and "harm." The "hurt" he is experiencing does not signify *harm* to his bones, joints and overall wellbeing and *the more active he is, the less pain he will feel*. This counterintuitive principle governs much of chronic pain treatment which exhorts patients to override their own protective impulses. Many and possibly most chronic pain patients develop *anticipatory fear of activities* they think will provoke their pain and become inactive. They fear and resist exercise though it will usually improve their pain through strengthening their muscles, reducing their mental stress and releasing endorphins. Exercise will also give patients self-efficacy, decrease *catastrophizing thoughts* and enable them to witness their own progress.

ALL THINGS ARE DIFFICULT BEFORE THEY ARE EASY

A few years ago, research was presented at a meeting of the American Academy of Pain Medicine that revealed how potent a force fear can be in pain patients. In a study conducted at Stanford University, Sean Mackey, M.D., Ph.D., Chief of the Pain Management found that "Those who had more fear during an acute low back pain episode were much more likely to ultimately overpredict the amount of pain they had, which ultimately led to significant increase in fear-avoidance behaviors, with subsequent worsening of symptoms, increase in duration of pain, and increase in disability (Frieden 2011)."

Dr. Mackey told participants that "catastrophizing has been found to be seven times more powerful than any other predictor in predicting the transition from acute to chronic pain."

For this reason, patients who have sustained injuries should be encouraged to return to their daily activities early, during the acute phase of healing, especially when X-rays show there are no fractures or serious problems. If acute pain is not properly managed or explained, patients can start to dwell on their pain which can often begin the path to chronic pain conditions. Medical professionals and the healthcare system in general can encourage this path through "enabling"—lenient time off work, kind attention, narcotics, and completing disability forms that provide financial remuneration. In countries in which there are not big financial settlements after accidents, recovery from chronic pain is often more swift and complete.

Clearly medical professionals who "baby" their patients by prescribing excessive rest, time off from work and "narcotics for pain" are not serving their long-term recovery or empowering them through helping them learn to control their pain and increase functioning at home and work.

Getting Started with a Pain Patient

Because pain is, by definition, subjective and can't be "proved," patients with chronic pain can suffer issues of "verifiability." They may feel that their pain is not being taken seriously by practitioners and even that they are suspecting of feigning pain for secondary gain, if litigation or worker compensation cases are ongoing. As medical professionals, it is not our job to judge the existence of pain—but to identify specific diagnoses and treatments and to gain a sense of the patient's narrative. Using a multidisciplinary approach facilitates acknowledging and *treating the "whole person" and not just "the pain."*

There is another way that chronic pain patients can feel ill-served by medical professionals. We know that pain is mediated by physiological pathways related to emotion, as well as, affected by cultural, vocational, and social factors. Unfortunately, patients can take this to mean that we think their pain is imaginary. When we tell them that their pain messages are linked to brain processes and emotional states, they can take this to mean the pain is somehow "in their head."

Ever since the publication of Ronald Melzack's *Gate Control Theory of Pain* in 1965, biomedical research has explored and confirmed the complex web of emotional, mental and cognitive processes behind the experience of pain. Dr. Melzack's groundbreaking Gate Theory and the other major pain theories are explored in depth in Chap. 3 of this book.

Studies have shown actual changes on functional MRI scans caused when cognitive modifications pertaining to pain were induced. When patients were prompted to view their pain in terms like "terrible," "horrible," and "incurable," the brain activity in their prefrontal cortex, a brain area that controls emotion and is linked to pain, increased. When the patients were instructed to pursue calm and pleasant thoughts through mind/body techniques, decreased pain activity was noted. Studies published on postoperative pain have shown that individuals who are more optimistic about their lives and the prospect of pain enjoy a better recovery and higher quality of life.

It is often human nature to "think the worst" and chronic pain patients are especially known to "catastrophize" their pain. Catastrophizing makes your patients' pain worse in two ways—it increases pain through *anticipation* of it and it limits activities that would distract them from their pain, causing them to focus on it more.

Focusing on pain also encourages patients to exhibit what are known as "pain behaviors" like verbal statements of pain or nonverbal pain behaviors like sighing, groaning, limping and grimacing. Just as research has revealed "acting happy" can produce feelings of happiness, enacting pain behaviors usually makes a patient feel worse. Pain behaviors *also invoke sympathy from family and caregivers which similarly can perpetuate the pain and disability "conviction."*

Because they are living intimately with a patient, family members are ideally included in treatment conferences as co-decision makers with valuable perspectives to offer. Family members exert major impacts on pain recovery. If they are focused on medicolegal aspects and specifically the hope of monetary settlements, a patient's pain behaviors can often be reinforced. When a family waits on a patient and excuses him of his household duties after weeks or months, it also reinforces the pain. However, if family members minimize or downplay a patient's pain, that is not an ideal situation either because feelings of self-pity and victimhood can be aroused. Notably, prescribing opioid painkillers can also perpetuate the patient and family's pain conviction by underscoring the belief that the pain must be considerable if it warrants opioid drugs.

The Brain/Pain Connection

Forgiveness does *not* change the past *but* it enlarges the future.
Patients should not focus on past mistreatment and anger at the doctors, employers, or insurers but *forgive*.

Like fear, anger has an augmentative effect on pain. If a patient's pain occurred due to someone else's fault such as in a motor vehicle accident or a work injury, he often harbors anger and even feelings of victimhood. "I was minding my business and look what happened to me," patients can intone to themselves over and over. If he is immersed in the medicolegal system, these emotions can be compounded if there are intense disagreements between insurance company doctors and his treating physician. Certainly insurance companies and attorneys are dedicated to the bottom line, not a patient's wellbeing which, unfortunately, adds to the volatility of the situation.

In addition to anger at their families and caregivers, chronic pain patients are often angry at their physicians and therapists, employers, and worker compensation authorities and insurance companies, who they feel are not helping the situation or making it worse. They can also be angry at *themselves* entertaining self-blaming thoughts like, "I should never have had that surgery" or "Why didn't I obtain a second opinion?"

While the convictions a patient holds about his pain, its causes and its prognosis, can add to his pain experience, these thoughts, sometimes called "self-talk," can also be controlled. Many patients can benefit from a method of self-inquiry like that developed by an American speaker and author Byron Katie, known for The Work (Katie 2014). She suggests four questions for people to pose when they are confronted with thoughts that cause them anger, fear, depression and addiction. (1) Is it true? (Yes or no. If no, move to (3)), (2) Can you absolutely know that it's true? (Yes or no), (3) How do you react emotionally, when you believe that thought?, and (4) Who would you be and what feelings would you have without the thought?

Questions to Apply to a Disturbing Thought

1. Is it true? (Yes or no. If no, move to (3))
2. Can you absolutely know that it's true? (Yes or no.)
3. How do you react, what happens, when you believe that thought?
4. Who would you be without the thought?

Byron Katie

The Work

There is also a strong relationship between pain and depression. Between 30 and 65 % of patients with chronic pain also have depression and studies have shown that patients who have depression and anxiety in addition to their pain, are 2–5 times more likely to develop chronic pain 1–8 years down the line (Frieden 2011). Sometimes, treating the underlying anxiety and depression can improve the patient's pain through the varied skills of the full multidisciplinary team. We will address emotion and mental factors involved in chronic pain more fully in Chap. 4 about Cognitive Behavioral treatments and Chap. 5, Treating the Chronic Pain Patient.

Even though a patient may have a clear "pain generator" causing nociceptive pain due to specific injury or medical condition such as recent back surgery or nerve damage, anxiety, depression and stress will frequently exacerbate the pain. The stressors of losing a job, mobility, independence and financial security can have profound effects on a patient's health in addition to the pain itself. Stress provokes the hypothalamic-pituitary-adrenocortical axis and hypothalamus to secrete cortisol and the sympathetic nervous system too increases the heart rate and stimulates the adrenal glands.

Stress often generates behavioral changes in a patient like increased smoking and drinking, increased or decreased sleep and decreased exercise and activities. It affects liver function, muscle tension, and the metabolism of food, facilitating weight gain.

Stress also leads to high levels of inflammation in the body and impairs the immune system itself—inviting more health problems.

Finally, several studies have identified traumatic and abusive events in the pasts of chronic pain patients which are triggered by the experience of pain as adults and add to their chronic pain situation (Finestone 2009).

Toward a New Attitude

Whether angry, stressed, resentful, fearful, self-critical, self-pitying or depressed, patients with chronic pain often benefit from a multidisciplinary approach that addresses both body and mind. Disappointed by months of ineffective treatments, they are often open to a new approach and willing to consider the idea, for the first time, that their pain will never be "cured" but can be managed in a way that they can still enjoy a high quality of life. Several books like *The Promise: Never Have Another Negative Thought Again* by Graham Price (Price 2013) chronicle this acceptance process which Price calls "pacceptance" for positive acceptance.

Many chronic pain patients, when they accept their pain, describe their ability to live successful lives despite recurrent or chronic pain as "the pain is no longer controlling me; I am controlling the pain." Sometimes an attitude shifts from "I am a pain patient who can do only a few things," to "I am a person who can do most things despite occasional pain." The change amounts to a Gestalt in their thinking; the patient has ceased "fighting" and accepted his condition in a new way.

Often the process of acceptance begins when a patient realizes, sometimes for the first time, that his pain and situation are no one's particular "fault." This allows built up anger to be redirected toward the positive motivation to improve and rebuild their lives. Even when a patient may not return to his former employment, pain patients can often identify new strengths and interests and their new lives can wind up preferable to their "pre-chronic pain lives." One of my patients was able to use his "season of suffering" with chronic pain to gain the training to become a health educator at the university level. Many pain patients are able to bring renewed affection to their families, especially spouses and children, when they reach a level of acceptance.

> Only if you have been in the deepest valley, can you ever know how magnificent it is to be on the highest mountain.
> Richard M. Nixon

While chronic pain patients who have not accepted their situation are very focused on "four-letter words" like "can't," "fear," and of course "pain," when they work with a multidisciplinary team and are educated in the mystery of pain, and techniques of self-management and self-efficacy, we often see a new word surfacing in their life: hope. I have discussed these issues in detail in my previous book, *Pain: A Four Letter Word You Can Live With—Understanding and controlling your pain* (Vasudevan 1995).

Even though it has been over 20 years since it was published, the principles in the book are true today.

In caring for patients with chronic pain for almost 40 years, I have been awed to see patients who were disabled by pain and dependent on narcotics and the health-care system change into vibrant, active people no longer debilitated by pain over a course of a short period of time. The main ingredient in these dramatic transformations is actually a *mixture* of all the ingredients found in multidisciplinary treatment including physical and psychological therapies, appropriate medications, education and the encouragement of a positive attitude of participation.

In her book *Positivity* Dr. Barbara L. Fredrickson (2009) describes such a change in attitude as a "tipping point," and uses the example of solid and rigid ice becoming flexible and flowing water under the right circumstances. Dr. Fredrickson notes that positive people tend to be healthier, happier and feel they have more control over their lives. Significantly, Dr. Fredrickson believes the quality of positivity can be learned.

The importance of positivity and living in the "now" is a theme that philosophers have addressed through the centuries. "If you are depressed you are living in the past; If you are anxious you are living in the future but if you are at peace you are living in the present," is an aphorism attributed to Lao Tzu. A more contemporary version of the thought is something I often say to my patients: "The past is history; the future is a mystery but today is a gift—that is why it is called the present."

There are many valuable books which seek to help patients uncover the spiritual aspects of their pain conditions often by modifying their attitudes and seeking "mindfulness." In spiritual communities such as Buddhist monasteries, mindfulness begins with the elimination of destructive thinking habits which produce stress and "striving" for an alert awareness and consciousness of thoughts and circumstances. For pain patients, being "mindful" translates into noting their own responses to pain and seeking to *choose* an attitude rather than have the pain control them.

In writing about the process in *A Mindfulness-Based Stress Reduction Workbook*, Bob Stahl, Ph.D. (Stahl 2010) declares that everyone has a choice in how to respond to situations. *If we are not aware we have a choice, we are often reenacting, old habitual patterns that may not really serve our health or wellbeing*, he suggests.

In his book, *Lead the Field*, Earl Nightingale (2002) emphasizes that positive attitude naturally translates into positive goal settings which lead to "true joy and satisfaction." He recounts an anecdote about a father who was trying to watch a football game while his young son frequently interrupted him. To keep the son busy, the father takes a newspaper with a photograph of the earth on it and tears the page into several pieces and throws it on the ground. Put "the world" back together, he suggests to his son, thinking it an impossible task and will keep the boy busy. Within a few minutes, the son has reconstructed the newspaper and returns to show it to his father. The father is rather amazed and asks the son how he accomplished it. The son replies, "On the back of the picture, there was a picture of a man and I put the man together and the world was put back together."

Impossible—It Is Just an opinion

Empowering the Pain Patient

The recovery of patients with chronic pain is often like that of alcoholics and addicts who, after proper interventions, can maintain their sobriety through supportive peer groups, family support and a commitment to a new attitude. The alcoholic will always be an alcoholic just like the chronic pain patient will always experience some pain. But both can choose their actions in light of their condition. Just as an alcoholic can choose to become a non-practicing alcoholic, a pain patient can choose to reject capitulation to pain and self-pity and apply what he has learned about his condition to good use and a productive life. It referring to the irreversibility of alcoholism, it is facetiously said in self-help groups, you can turn a cucumber into a pickle, but you cannot turn the pickle back into a cucumber. Still "you can be a great pickle." The same bittersweet observation applies to chronic pain patients.

Just as non-drinking alcoholics learn how to cope with the "triggers" that in the past made them want to pour a drink, pain patients can learn appropriate psychological techniques to "turn down the volume" of their pain and decrease their attention to it. In the Cognitive Behavioral approaches you will learn in Chap. 4, you can assist your patients in learning relaxation techniques and other mechanisms based on understanding their pain, using rational thinking about the pain and problem solving.

For example, when a chronic pain patient is having a flare up of pain he can say to himself, I *feel* like going to the emergency room—but I *know* that all I will get is more X-rays and more medication and it will not get to the source of my pain, because it never has!" This is what alcoholics would call "thinking through the drink." Instead, the pain patient uses self-management techniques he has learned that have worked in the past such as heat, muscle relaxation, and mental techniques. In this way, the chronic pain patient "resists" giving in to his pain the way an alcoholic resists taking a drink.

There is another concept in self-help groups for alcoholics which is to try the new approach and if it doesn't work "your misery will be refunded." Certainly most pain patients would not want their disability, dysfunction, drug misuse, and deconditioning "refunded." Nor will most pain patients fail to appreciate that insanity is "doing the same thing over and over again and expecting different results." More than most patients medical professionals see, pain patients realize if they keep doing what they have been doing, they will keep "getting what they have been getting."

This tipping point in which a pain patient has a new attitude of acceptance and positivity does not happen in a vacuum. It is the result of appropriate education, supportive staff, multidisciplinary specialists, supportive family and the patient's willingness and self-motivation to leave behind a life of dependency on the health-care system and drugs for a more functional lifestyle. The patient who was seeking a cure ends up with a different and more effective type of cure—from Commitment, Understanding, Resources and Empowerment as seen in Table 2.7.

Table 2.7 A "cure" pain patients can administer to themselves

C—Commitment. The engine behind the desire to want to get better
U—Understanding. Learn about pain conditions and management options
R—Resources. Primary care physicians, physical and occupational therapists, psychologists, and others
E—Empowerment. Being a team member and co-decision maker in treatments

When it comes to overcoming chronic pain, patients can be like caterpillars: there is nothing initially to indicate there is a butterfly in the making. Pain patients can also be thought of as seeds and we clinicians are the gardeners. Every seed or acorn has an internal compass that tells it when it has the ideal conditions in which to germinate. Until the seed senses that it is enveloped with the right moisture and soil nutrients, air temperature, and amount of sunlight, nothing can make it to sprout and it may be dormant for years. However, when the right soil, air and weather conditions are present, practically nothing can *stop* the seed from germinating and turn into the plant or tree it was programmed to become (Table 2.8).

Table 2.8 Main points of this chapter

Both patients and physicians lack knowledge about chronic pain
Chronic pain is not just biomedical it is biopsychosocial
Multidisciplinary care is more effective than unimodal treatments with chronic pain
Acute and chronic pain require different treatment approaches
Overuse of diagnostic imagery creates false positives and patient stress
The attitude of the patient is the key determinant of a positive pain outcome getting off

Getting off on the right foot with your chronic pain patient calls for skills that many of us do not use when we are treating patients with acute conditions. Chapter 6, Treating the Chronic Pain Patient, Chap. 9, Common Pain Problems, Low Back Pain and Chap. 10, Common Pain Problems, Complex Regional Pain Syndrome, Myofascial Syndrome, and Fibromyalgia address treatment of your chronic pain patient in depth.

References

American Academy of Pain Medicine. (2011). *Incidence of pain, as compared to major conditions*. Chicago: American Academy of Pain Medicine.

Debar, L. L., Kindler, L., Keefe, F. J., Green, C. A., Smith, D. H., Deyo, R. A., et al. (2012). A primary care-based interdisciplinary team approach to the treatment of chronic pain utilizing a pragmatic clinical trials framework. *Translational Behavioral Medicine, 2*(4), 523–530.

Fauber, J. (2012, October 2). Many injured workers remain on opioids, study finds. *Milwaukee Journal Sentinel.*

Fauber, J. & Gabler, E. (2012, May 30). Narcotic painkiller use booming among elderly. *Milwaukee Journal Sentinel/Medpage.*

Finestone, H. (2009). *The pain detective.* Santa Barbara, CA: Paeger.

Fishman, S. (2012a). *Listening to pain* (p. 67). Oxford, England: Oxford University Press.

Fishman, S. (2012b). *Responsible opioid prescribing.* Washington, DC: Waterford Life Sciences.

Fishman, S. (2014). *Model policy for the use of opioid analgesics in the treatment of chronic pain.* Washington, DC: Federation of State Medical Boards.

Fredrickson, B. (2009). *Positivity.* New York: Harmony Books.

Frieden, J. (2011, March 28). AAPM: State of mind can turn acute pain to chronic. *Medpage Today.*

Frost, R. (2002). *The road not taken: A selection of Robert Frost's poems.* New York: Owl Books.

Groopman, J. (2007). *How doctors think* (p. 181). New York: Houghton Mifflin.

Hadler, N. (2009). *Stabbed in the back* (p. 44). Chapel Hill: University of North Carolina Press.

Hanscom, D. (2012). *Back in control.* Seattle, WA: Vertus Press.

Institute of Medicine. (2011). *Relieving pain in America* (p. 11). Washington, DC: The National Academies Press.

International Association for the Study of Pain. (2012). Interdisciplinary chronic pain management: International perspectives. *Pain Clinical Updates, 20,* 7.

International Association for the Study of Pain (2013, June). *Insight,* pp. 19–20. New York: Academies Press.

Katie, B. (2014). *The work of Byron Katie.* Retrieved from http://www.thework.com/index.php

McAllister, M. J., McKenzie, K. E., Schultl, D. M., & Epshteyn, M. G. (2005). Effectiveness of a multidisciplinary chronic pain program for treatment of refractory patients with complicated chronic pain syndromes. *Pain Physician, 8*(4), 369–373.

Moradi, B., Hagmann, S., Zahlten-Hinguranage, A., Caldeira, F., Putz, C., Rosshirt, N., et al. (2012). Efficacy of multidisciplinary treatment for patients with chronic low back pain: A prospective clinical study in 395 patients. *Journal of Clinical Rheumatology, 18*(2), 76–82.

Nightingale, E. (2002). *Lead the field.* New York: Simon & Schuster.

Price, G. (2013). *The promise: Never have another negative thought again.* London, England: Pearson Education Limited.

Ochoa, G. (2012, April). Pain education lacking in medical schools. *Pain Medicine News.*

Rasmussen, C., Nielsen, G. L., Hansen, V. K., Jensen, O. K., & Schioettz-Christensen, B. (2005). Rates of lumbar disc surgery before and after implementation of multidisciplinary nonsurgical spine clinics. *Spine, 30*(21), 2469–2473.

Stahl, B. (2010). *A mindfulness-based stress reduction workbook.* Oakland, CA: New Harbinger.

Vasudevan, S. (1995). *Pain: A four letter word you can live with—Understanding and controlling your pain.* Milwaukee, WI: Montgomery Media.

Webster, L. (2013, August). 'We have an epidemic on our hands and the status quo is failing us': an interview with Lynn Webster, MD. *Pain Medicine News.*

Wells-Federman, C. L. (1999). Care of the patient with chronic pain: Part I. *Clinical Excellence for Nurse Practitioners, 3*(4), 192–204.

Chapter 3
Major Pain Theories and Factors Behind Chronic Pain

In all of medicine there may be no bigger mystery than chronic, nonmalignant pain—especially to those of us who treat it. Pain usually serves a biological purpose, yet in chronic pain patients, pain symptoms seem to exist with little biologically useful purpose. We know that pain can be ignored by soldiers and first responders in crises, yet chronic pain improbably exists in limbs that are amputated or paralyzed. We know that pain that is considered debilitating in one culture can be barely acknowledged in another culture. And finally we know the same pain event that resolves in one patient can turn into chronic pain with its associated debilitating features in another.

These ambiguities and even paradoxes in the experience of pain, seen in Table 3.1, strain the physician/pain patient relationship as both parties become frustrated at the ability of chronic pain to confound treatment.

Pain is derived from the word Pu which is Sanskrit for "sacrifice" and Peon, a Latin word that means "punishment." In written literature, chronic pain dates back at least as far as the Bible in which Jeremiah says "Why is my pain perpetual, and my wound incurable [which] refuseth to be healed? (King James 1611). It is clear that even hundreds of years ago, chronic pain had a strong emotional component.

Clearly pain is necessarily to our survival. In rare cases, humans are born without the ability to encode and process harmful stimuli in the nervous system (nociception) and endure dangerous consequences. Medical textbooks tell the story of "Miss C." a Canadian girl who was born with a congenital insensitivity to pain (Melzack and Wall 1982). Miss C. "showed no physiological changes in response to noxious stimuli. Similarly she never sneezed or coughed, had an extremely weak gag reflex, and no corneal reflex. As a child, Miss C. bit off the tip of her tongue and sustained third-degree burns from her inability to sense pain (Melzack and Wall 1982, p. 4). As an adult, she developed severe erosion and infection in her knees, hip and spine from failing to shift her weight or turn over in bed known as "Charcot joint." Eventually, her insensitivity to pain took her life though "careful study of her nervous system showed no abnormalities."

© Springer International Publishing Switzerland 2015
S. Vasudevan, *Multidisciplinary Management of Chronic Pain*,
DOI 10.1007/978-3-319-20322-5_3

Table 3.1 Puzzles of pain

The paradoxes in pain management include	
Most pain serves a biological useful purpose to the person and clinician	Chronic pain doesn't serve a useful biological purpose
Severe pain can be ignored in a crisis	Pain can exist in paralyzed or amputated limbs
Pain is minimized in some cultures	Pain is emphasized in some cultures
Some patients fully recover from pain	Some patients never fully recover and have chronic pain

In other instances of congenital insensitivity to pain, patients have developed bone fractures and deformities and infections of the tongue, lips, gums, eye, bones and joints because of their imperviousness to pain. Unable to feel heat, cold or even the need to urinate, these patients often injure themselves due to their lack of pain messages. They have even been known to develop syndromic mental retardation from hyperthermia in hot weather because of their inability to sweat (Sayyahfar et al. 2013).

Yet is also clear that pain perception can be "turned off" in some instances. In parts of India, in an ancient agricultural ritual that is still practiced, villagers hang from hooks embedded in their backs to bless children and crops, yet show no sign of pain (Melzack and Wall 1982, p. 16). In Africa, India and other places, trepanation, a type of primitive brain surgery, is still practiced without painkillers and no outward appearance of distress on the part of the patients. Trepanation involves drilling a hole or more into a patient's skull to allow air to enter and relieve intracranial pressure seen with intracranial diseases. Even though the brain does not have pain fibers, the skull certainly does. Yet this procedure is, amazingly, performed without apparent pain.

Certainly, we see other instances of the variations in pain expression that are influenced by a patient's past experience, state of mind, expectations, culture, family, and the "meaning" ascribed to the pain. One of the best examples is childbirth which women endure and repeat for the obvious benefit at the end. Childbirth is so painful, it is said facetiously, that if men had to go through it, the human species would "die out."

Actually, memory of pain can have two distinct characters in human beings. Often, we can't recall and reexperience some of our most past excruciatingly painful experiences which is why it is said that "pain has no memory." However, some patients, paradoxically, reproduce and reexperience memories of pain, including certain emotions associated with an event, despite healing of their biophysical pain. This is sometimes seen when trying to treat patients with Post-Traumatic Stress Disorders (PTSD) or childhood abuse experiences or memories.

As we noted in Chap. 1 of this book, current medical science cannot fully explain how pain "happens" or the etiology of chronic pain conditions. Nevertheless, we will examine the main theories of pain, shown in Table 3.2, which have shaped and continue to shape current medicine practice.

Table 3.2 Leading theories of pain

Door Bell Theory
Gate Theory
Mismatch Theory
Loeser Model of Pain
Chemical Theory
Learning Theory
Social/Cultural Modeling Theory
Social and Legal Theory
Psychological Factors Theory
Matrix Theory of pain
Spinal Cord Mechanisms
Brain-Based Pain Modulation
Neuroimmune Interactions
Pain Genetics

The Door Bell Theory

The Door Bell Theory, which dates back to 1644, contends that when the "door bell" of pain rings, it means a pain generator is at the door. Well recognized by patients and medical professionals, The Door Bell Theory is likely the most common theory of pain and it is certainly useful in most acute situations. Yet the theory fails to explain much chronic pain, in which there is often no specific injury and no one at the "door," such as in patients with migraine headaches, fibromyalgia or pain after shingles. Eighty percent of patients with migraines, for example, have no discernible "injury." Nor does a pain "visitor" always ring the bell. Also, almost everyone has had the experience of cutting themselves, perhaps cooking or gardening, and not realizing it until they see the blood, because they felt no pain. Not too long ago, my wife injured her arm while gardening. X-rays revealed the arm was broken in seven different places yet she reported that her pain on a 1–10 scale was a 2 or 3.

Despite its shortcomings, the Door Bell Theory describes a good warning system which is usually helpful to the patient and physician in understanding some sources of pain and setting up a treatment plan. But when the door bell is "faulty," and no one is at the door, the message to convey to your patients is that they should stop *opening* the door and responding to the door bell. Patients can effectively learn to ignore a "faulty door bell" and to stop seeking answers in the healthcare system and to stop undergoing numerous, unnecessary tests.

Also, as we have noted elsewhere in this book, there is no one-to-one correlation between pain and injury or pain and abnormalities shown on X-rays and other diagnostic imagery, as this theory would imply. Many or even most chronic pain patients lack a clear injury to explain their pain and a pain generator is seldom disclosed on common medical tests. While X-rays and MRI and CT scans are increasingly used to hone in on the patient's pain, as well as functional nerve tests and other lab diagnostics, a pain generator is rarely revealed. The dismaying truth about conditions ranging from joint pain, neck pain, headaches, and some spinal conditions to fibromyalgia, complex regional pain syndromes and lower back pain is: the source of the pain is often not identified with today's sophisticated imagery.

As we saw in the previous chapter, scans often will reveal abnormalities but they are frequently not the pain generator. Patients can end up treated for these identified abnormalities while the source of their pain is not addressed. Patients can also be subject to undue and unnecessary stress when treated for abnormalities that were likely not the cause of their pain. In our current healthcare system, expensive technology is overused, resulting in patients who are overscreened and overdiagnosed for conditions which "nature" and time would likely have resolved. Overscreening is so widespread, patients can feel like they did not receive top medical care if their injury was not X-rayed and given other diagnostic imaging and physicians can cater to this (mis)perception. Such "misattribution" leads to treating the condition shown on the MRI or the X-ray and not the person with pain, as other causes are not evaluated and treated.

Of course imaging technology is invaluable for *acute pain* which is treated very differently. Unlike chronic pain, acute pain usually resolves in 2–6 weeks with rest, time and physical therapy, injections and medications as needed.

As the philosophical pendulum has swung back from a multidisciplinary model of pain to a biological one, clinicians assume there must be underlying disease or a tissue injury when a patient complains of pain or demonstrates "pain behaviors" and they seek a pain generator. This is one of the hazards of unimodal and uncoordinated approaches to pain, versus multidisciplinary care; practitioners treat the pain and not the patient and even "read and treat the X-ray" instead of "reading and treating the patient." Yet chronic pain can seldom, if ever, be effectively treated without taking into consideration a patient's psychological, cultural, environmental, social and legal milieu.

The Gate Theory

The Gate Theory was considered revolutionary when described in 1965 by Melzack and Wall. It proposes that stimulation of innocuous neural pathways, carried on the large myelinated A-fibers can block concurrent noxious information carried from the smaller, C- fibers. Signals from the A-fibers, carrying information about touch, temperature, pressure, and electrical sensations, can "close the gate" on the C-fibers which carry pain messages to the spinal cord and then to the brain, by preempting them, according to this theory. It is postulated that this happens through direct inhibition of pain transmission in the dorsal horn of the spinal cord and possible recruitment of endogenous inhibitory pathways through the columns of the spinal cord.

We now know that emotional states like anxiety, depression, frustration, fear, and anger (often related to a work injury or car accident) usually open the "gates." Conversely, the gate is often "closed" by exercise, heat, cold, pressure, psychological approaches such as Cognitive Behavior Therapy (CBT), Acceptance and Commitment Therapy (ACT), relaxation and stress reduction techniques and some medications. Electrical stimulation, whether peripheral stimulation such as transcutaneous electrical nerve stimulation (TENS) or spinal cord stimulation (SCS) are also known to close the gate, as are psychological techniques such as relaxation, positive thinking and mind-body techniques. Many of these techniques are discussed in Chap. 4, about Cognitive Behavioral Therapy (CBT) techniques.

The Mismatch Theory

This theory postulates that the brain has the ability to modify and completely suppress pain for short periods of time. A demonstration of the theory would be enacted when someone's received a cup of coffee that is too hot to hold. While the normal biological response would be to immediately drop the cup, according to this theory, the brain can recognize a "mismatch" in a situation—perhaps the cup holder is at a boss' house or exclusive facility where it would not be appropriate to simply drop the cup—therefore the person can override the impulse. Instead, the brain can inform the hand *not* to drop the hot cup but to walk a few steps and find an acceptable place to put it.

Central to the Mismatch Theory is that when the brain is continually told to overcome pain recognition and the pain cannot be overcome, the patient experiences anxiety, frustration, anger, helplessness, and hopelessness. We often see that aggregation of emotions in patients with many chronic pain conditions, especially those with fibromyalgia, where there is a "sensory amplification" leading to a wide spectrum of symptoms not explainable by pathological nociception.

One alternative chronic pain treatment that employs the Mismatch Theory is Mirror Therapy. In one study at Bath Royal National Hospital for Rheumatic Diseases, healthy volunteers seated in front of mirrors that made them look symmetrical, hiding one arm, were asked to move their arms on the basis of their reflection, creating a "mismatch" between the actual motion and mirror motion (Vince 2005). "Almost instantly they began to feel sensations in the arm they couldn't see," said Candy McCabe of the University of Bath in the United Kingdom. Under this theory, subjects' brains were "correcting" the mismatch.

In another study, eight patients with Complex Regional Pain Syndrome (CRPS) were seated in front of mirrors such that their painful limb was occluded and they appeared to have two health arms. After being instructed to "try to believe" the mirror depiction, patients experienced pain relief, in some cases, instantly. When the mirror was removed, the pain returned, said researchers. CRPS is discussed in depth in Chap. 10 of this book.

When we explain to patients that pain is "in their brain," they can wrongfully deduce that we mean it is imaginary or "in the mind," This theory provides strong evidence of the brain's perceptual role in the experience of pain. The Mismatch Theory is also useful in conveying to patients who say they have "no control" over pain that control *is possible* even for few seconds. It is noteworthy that when patients begin to improve from chronic pain, they frequently change their conviction say they are no longer "controlled" by their pain.

The Loeser Model

The Loeser Model of pain, proposed by John Loeser of the University of Washington, Seattle more than three decades ago, construes the pain experience as four layers, seen in Fig. 3.1 and Table 3.3, or "onion rings," which move outward from physical factors to behavioral factors.

At the center Loeser's "onion" are the physiological factors of nociception as described in the Door Bell Theory. Yet, as the layers move outward, the pain experience becomes increasingly subjective from the actual quality of pain that patients try to share with us to their interpretation of the sensations ("Suffering") and their bodily responses ("Pain Behavior").

At the heart of Loeser's theory is the recognition that, while a patient's pain may not be resolvable, his behaviors can lessen his pain if the patient is willing and able to replace them with "well" behaviors. This constitutes the goal of therapy under the Loeser model—to decrease the suffering and pain behaviors—and replace them with "well behaviors."

Loeser's theory also acknowledges that the degree of suffering a patient's experiences often encompasses his predictions of what the pain "means" medically, and is

Fig. 3.1 The loeser model of pain

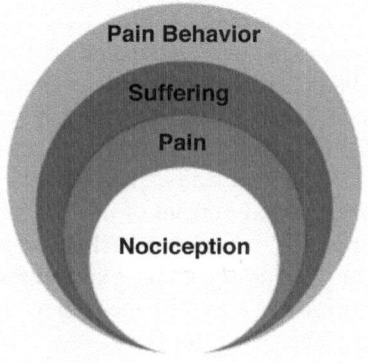

Table 3.3 The Loeser four layers of pain

Nociception	Chemical, thermal, and mechanical factors irritation of nerves (injury/tissue damage)
Pain	An unpleasant sensory and emotional experience associated with tissue damage and emotional activation
Suffering	Emotional response triggered by nociception that includes fear, anxiety, depression, and hopelessness
Pain Behavior	Verbal/nonverbal expressions such as grimacing, limping or avoiding activities that convey to the outside world the patient is in pain

also affected by his culture. For example, patients know that pain after they exercise and certainly during childbirth is "normal." Yet other pain is often regarded as harmful, especially if it is unfamiliar. *It is important that we explain to patients the difference between "hurt" (which implies pain) and "harm" (which implies further damage or injury) as we noted in the last chapter.*

A depiction of how the Loeser theory of pain translates into treatment is found in Chap. 8, Creating a Multidisciplinary Team. In almost 40 years of seeing and treating chronic pain patients, Loeser's theory has been of immense value to me—as it has been to my colleagues.

The Chemical Theory

The Chemical Theory postulates that neurotransmitters such as prostaglandin, P substance, aldolase, glutamate, serotonin, norepinephrine, endorphin, and GABA are behind much chronic pain. It is often noted that in patients with sensory amplification syndromes like fibromyalgia (in which abnormal processing of sensations can make sounds appear louder, lights brighter and smells more acute) it seems their "nerves are having a seizure." As clinicians began to prescribe antiseizure drugs like gabapentin (Neurontin) and pregabalin (Lyrica), approved by FDA for neuropathic pain, and several other antiseizure drugs used empirically, the nerve "seizures" of these patients improved. Several antidepressant drugs are used to modify chemicals in the brain to decrease pain, associated depression and insomnia like the tricyclics amitriptyline and nortriptyline and the serotonin norepinephrine reuptake inhibitor (SNRI) drugs like duloxetine (Cymbalta) and milnacipran (Savella). The fact that these drugs are effective with neuropathic pain, pain caused by the dysfunction or disease/injury of nerves, and in "sensory amplification syndromes" such as fibromyalgia lends credibility to the Chemical Theory.

In addition to treatment with tricyclic and SNRI medications, patients whose pain is neuropathic often improve with exercise and CBT and psychological approaches. These modalities can have similar modulating effects on neurotransmitters as the medications dampen pain. We explore pharmaceutical treatments in Chap. 6 and CBT and psychological approaches in Chap. 4.

The Learning Theory

The Learning Theory hypothesizes that a behavior that is punished will tend to be extinguished and behavior that is rewarded will tend to be reinforced and recur. Certainly, punishing unwanted human behavior, whether exceeding the speed limit or committing violence, is a basic legal tenet of civilization. Yet there are also limitations to how well the principles of creating "negative consequence" as part of the Learning Theory induce sustained changes in behavior. Despite knowing the negative consequences of smoking, overeating and failure to exercise, patients continue to do all three! Some patients will refrain from these habits for a short period of time—while they are on an airplane or in the hospital—but then resume them later. Still, positive reinforcement of "well behaviors" and negative reinforcement, including ignoring, of "pain behaviors" that do not serve a biologically useful function, has been a major tenet of multidisciplinary pain rehabilitation programs and a main reason for their success.

There are many aspects of contemporary pain treatment that can reward and reinforce a patient's pain from time off work and long-term narcotics to the sympathetic attention of medical staff and family members. Unlike the situation in most countries, pain patients in the United States often await prospective financial settlements from accidents or on-the-job injuries. Financial settlements certainly do not reward the patient's "well" or pain-free behavior. In Australia, work-related disorders like carpal tunnel syndrome reached almost "epidemic proportions," according to a study, until the government reclassified the conditions as no longer work-related. Then, the number of complaints by individuals of carpal tunnel-like symptoms dramatically decreased (Fink 1997).

Yet positive learning is also possible with chronic pain patients. When patients become active members of their treatment team, making a commitment to exercise and lifestyle alterations, pursuing psychological guidance when necessary, educating themselves about chronic pain and attempting to develop a new "attitude," they receive reinforcements from their clinicians and rewards in their personal life. As we noted in the previous chapter, patients with chronic pain face similar recovery features of alcoholics and addicts. If they make a commitment to a new lifestyle, it becomes its own reward and they would seldom consider returning to their previous lifestyle.

Social or Cultural Modeling

Over the decades of my practice, I have noted that every pain patient who comes to our offices brings to the visit five unique "B's": biography, beliefs, biology, behavior and bodily response—which are interrelated, shown in Table 3.4.

Table 3.4 The "B's"

Biography	What is patient's story? Background?
Beliefs	What does pain mean to him?
Biology	How physiology is affected?
Behavior	What are verbal/nonverbal behaviors?
Bodily response	What are responses to pain, inactivity, disability, and interventions?

Response to pain is learned from familial environments in which children witness their parents' and family members' reactions or attitudes to pain. For example, in one study children's pain thresholds were altered by exposure to their mother's behavior (Goodman and McGrath 2003).

Pain memories can persist in pain patients from their childhood (Henry 2011). Painful procedures *received as a neonate* resulted in abnormal central nervous system responses to pain in adults in one study in a 2010 study in the journal *Pain*. These pain memories can be "influenced by psychological interventions such as operant and classical conditioning," writes Henry.

In addition to affecting the patient separately, the five B's also are cyclical and affect each other. Just as a patient's biography and how he was raised, affects his beliefs, his biography and beliefs affect the health care he seeks and receives. The treatment a patient receives, in turn, affects his bodily responses, behavior, and biography. It is probably fair to say that, like a mobile, it is not possible to alter one "B" of the five Bs without altering all of them. The B's constitute a subtle, intertwined system that determines both who a patient is and how he lives with and regards his pain. The more accurately a medical professional can perceive and respect this complex matrix, the better care we can give.

Certainly, we know from many studies that cultural philosophies toward pain are major determinants of individual pain reactions. In *The War on Pain*, Scott Fishman notes that at one time in Lithuania there were few complaints of neck pain or "whiplash" after motor vehicle collisions because "there was no legal system in place in which an individual could sue for damages resulting from a car accident" (Fishman and Berger 2001). The medical literature offers many cross-cultural examples of the experience of pain and its diversity.

Social and Legal Theories

As we touched on under the Learning Theory, when a patient is injured at work, the Workers' Compensation system can become an active force in his treatment and recovery. While a majority of patients with work injuries who get appropriate treatment, return to work with no permanent disability or litigation, 5–10 % do not. This small percentage of patients who do not improve under the Workers' Compensation system accounts for over 90 % of the expenses in the system in almost every state.

In these instances, the Workers' Compensation system and/or a patient's employer or the medicolegal system in motor vehicle accidents, can become barriers to his recovery.

If a motor vehicle accident is behind what a patient believes is causing his pain, there can also be extenuating factors that block recovery. The patient often feels wronged and desires compensation for his suffering which sparks two emotions, self-pity and anger, that are known to exacerbate pain. Families can also reinforce this pain, if they become litigious and self-righteous. When a patient is an accident victim, he can become a pawn in a financially based game with his lawyer and physician on one side and insurance company lawyers and other physicians on the other. This situation will usually exacerbate his pain. We will explore disability and related issues in Chap. 7.

Psychological Factors

As we noted in the last chapter, up to 65 % of patients with chronic pain also have depression. When a patient has depression and anxiety in addition to his pain, his pain is much more likely to become chronic according to studies (Frieden 2011). Moreover, the fact of his changed lifestyle, often devoid of work and activities and people he used to enjoy, adds to the depressed state as do other emotions which are common both in people with chronic pain and depression. Studies have demonstrated that anger, whether at a patient's employer, family, his medical practitioners or an insurance company, usually increases pain. Fear has similar effects on pain which is why anticipatory fear—trepidation about activities that could reignite pain—should be addressed in pain patients. When patients are willing to risk activities which they are afraid will ignite their pain, often working with multidisciplinary practitioners, their pain often begins to dissipate and they start the road to recovery.

Finally, pain patients will usually improve if they can grasp the attitude of acceptance—accepting that their pain will likely never disappear but they can have a high quality of life despite occasional pain. *Acceptance is a "master" emotion that mediates many other emotions and often marks a turning point in recovery.*

The Matrix/Neuromatrix Theory

Ronald Melzack, Ph.D., who along with Patrick Wall proposed the Gate Theory of pain in 1965, made important contributions to the understanding of the central nervous system (CNS) as contributing to the understanding of pain. In 1999, Dr. Melzack noted that the Gate Theory forced the medical and biological sciences to accept the brain as an active system that filters, selects, and modulates inputs to the CNS (Melzack 1999). He emphasized that the dorsal horns of the spinal cord are not

Table 3.5 Multiple inputs in the neuromatrix theory

1. Sensory inputs from skin and organs
2. Visual and other inputs affecting cognitive interpretation
3. Cognitive and emotional inputs from other areas of the brain
4. The inhibitory modulation of all brain functions
5. Stress regulatory areas including chemical, endocrine, immune factors, and individual genetic composition

merely passive transmission stations but have dynamic activities where inhibition, excitation, and modulation occur. He proposed that the brain possessed a network of nerves, called the body-self-neuromatrix—which integrates multiple inputs to produce an output pattern that evokes pain sensation. This network includes the ability to be sensory-discriminative, affective-motivational and to evaluative-cognitive dimensions of the pain experience. According to this theory, as we see in Table 3.5, the multiple inputs that act with the neuromatrix programs include:

1. Sensory inputs from the skin, organs, and other somatic receptors
2. Visual and other sensory inputs that influence our cognitive interpretation
3. Cognitive and emotional inputs from other areas of the brain
4. The inhibitory modulation of all brain functions
5. The body's stress regulatory areas including chemical, endocrine (hormonal), immune and opioid systems of the body, along with the genetic composition of the person.

The Neuromatrix Theory encompasses numerous interrelations between body systems and functions in contradistinction to the "one-to-one relationship" between an injury/pain generator and the pain experience. It both sums up many of the previously mentioned theories and clearly demonstrates the complexity of the pain process which makes it not amenable to the simplistic peripheral philosophy of pain. *The theory also raises questions of the unimodality approaches, especially interventional or pharmacologic approaches used in isolation.*

Mosely, in a paper titled "A pain neuromatrix approach to patients with chronic pain," provides an approach to rehabilitation of patients with pain using this theoretical basis (Moseley 2003). This paper emphasizes that: (1) pain is an output of the brain that is produced whenever the brain concludes that body tissue is in danger and action is required and (2) pain is a multisystem output that is produced when an individual-specific neuromatrix is activated. The treatment focuses on decreasing all inputs that convey the body is in danger and activating components of the pain neuromatrix *without activating its outputs*. The multidisciplinary treatment model, with its emphasis on empowering patients about "what is right with them" as opposed to "what is wrong with them" is well suited to this approach. The neuromatrix theory provides some insight into why patients with chronic pain may have little or no discernable injury/pain generator and why psychological, social, and stressful input can trigger the experience of chronic pain.

Spinal Cord Mechanisms

As we learned with the Gate Control Theory, the main gateway for pain in the CNS is the dorsal horn. But, scientists are increasingly learning, the "gate" is not a simple relay station as once envisioned but a complex "circuit" where peripheral sensations are transducted, transmitted, and modulated by the brain's descending fibers which either can excite or diminish the activity in this circuit of nerves which are in constant communication.

The communication is mediated through numerous chemicals including N-methyl-D-aspartate (NMDA), glutamate receptors which are excitatory, gamma amino butyric acid (GABA) receptors and glycine receptors which are inhibitory. Small nerve cells in the dorsal horn of the spinal cord called microglia are involved in these interactions and modify the activity of the nerve transmission up to the brain. A "soup" of chemicals including G-protein, GABA, adenosine, substance P, calcitonin gene-related peptide (CGRP), opioid receptors and several ion channels are involved in exciting or inhibiting the transmission of pain. Thus the spinal cord, rather than a passive "transfer station" of pain and other sensations is robust and active with several neurotransmitters interacting to produce the pain experience.

These spine mechanisms seem to explain why many patients, especially with neuropathic or chronic pain, will complain of pain after a stimulus is withdrawn. This summation of overexcited nerves leads to a process called "wind-up"—the increase of nociceptive pain perception without an injury. This increased nerve responsiveness to minimally painful nociceptive stimuli is due to the plasticity of the CNS and called "central sensitization." It is a hallmark of many chronic pain syndromes.

Another way the spinal cord is more involved with chronic pain than previously believed relates to glial cells. For years these cells were considered inactive and serving only as scaffolding for other grey matter but it is now believed microglia, the smallest of the glial cells, can induce neuroinflammation, hyperarousal of the sympathetic nervous system (SNS), and stimulation of the hypothalamic-pituitary complex, thus causing and maintaining neuropathic pain (Tennant 2014). This may explain why antiseizure drugs like gabapentin (Lyrica), gabanergic drugs such as baclofen or tizanidine and antidepressants like duloxetine (Cymbalta) and amitriptyline are often effective in chronic pain syndromes characterized by central sensitization.

Brain-Based Pain Modulation

In the past two decades, advances in neuroimaging techniques like electroencephalography (EEG), positron emission tomography (PET), and functional magnetic resonance imaging (fMRI) have provided a better understanding of the role of the primary (S1) and secondary (S2), somatosensory areas of the brain in pain. They have also shed light on the role of the limbic system in pain which includes the anterior cingulate cortex (ACC), prefrontal cortex, insula, amygdala, thalamus, ventral tegmental areas, and cerebellum.

It is the involvement of these areas of the brain (which also control mood and motivation) in the pain process that makes me tell my patients "pain is in the brain." Far from suggesting a patient's pain is imaginary, brain-based theories of pain mean the brain processes pain perception including a *patient's expectations*, *experience*, *and the prevailing environmental factors* (Coghill et al 2003; Koyama et al. 2005). The latter effects are why psychological treatments such as CBT, are effective as we discuss in Chap. 4.

Early evidence for brain-based pain modulatory mechanisms came from observations of H.K. Beecher, a physician who served with the United States Army during the Second World War (Ossipov and Porreca 2014). Beecher noted when soldiers were in combat situations, they could experience a remarkable attenuation of pain. As many as three-quarters of badly wounded soldiers reported no to moderate pain and did not want pain relief medication, he observed—though the wounds were major and consisted of compound fractures of long bones or penetrating wounds of the abdomen, thorax, or cranium. Moreover, only individuals who were clearly alert, responsive, and not in shock were included in his report leading to the conclusion that "strong emotions" block pain (Ossipov and Porreca 2014). Analogous observations have been seen in others, including athletes who continue competition despite significant injuries.

This theory, which accords with the Neuromatrix Theory in which the pattern of activity of interconnected regions and the interplay of inhibitory and excitatory systems modulates pain experience, also provides an understanding of the motivational aspects of pain such as conditioned pain modulation (CPM), negative learned behaviors, and opioid habituation because they are controlled by related descending noradrenergic inhibition. Certainly, less efficient CPM has been demonstrated in irritable bowel syndrome (IBS), fibromyalgia, osteoarthritis, rheumatoid arthritis, interstitial cystitis (IC), post-herpetic neuralgia, and chronic tension/migraine headaches—all central centalization syndromes involving dysfunctional endogenous pain-modulating systems. These findings go a long way in explaining why physical therapy approaches, psychological approaches that modify motivation, cognition, and mood and medications that modulate the descending spinal cord pathways are proving so effective in chronic pain.

Neuroimmune Interactions

While several types of cells contribute to the chemical environment of chronic pain conditions, there is considerable evidence that peripheral immune cells play a key role. In a review of neuroimmune interactions involved in pain, Bennett et al. describe the ways in which the immune system can alter sensory perception and cause or maintain persistent pain. Cytokines and chemokines, they write, not only act as mediators of pain but are involved in "peripheral sensitization of nociceptors" (Bennett et al. 2014).

The neuroimmune theory seems to explain why drugs which block tumor necrosis factors (TNF), interleukin-1β (IL-1β), nerve growth factor (NGF), the chemokines CCL2, CCL3, CCL4, CCL7, CCL11, CXCL1, CXCL2, CXCL4, CXCL7, and CXCL8 and oral and topical NSAIDs can be effective in pain treatment: they modulate peripheral immune mechanisms involved in inflammation (Dawes et al. 2011).

Similarly centrally neuroimmune interactions and microglia have been implicated in neuropathic pain states and complex regional pain syndromes. This developing theory provides the rationale for using glucocorticoids (steroids), intravenous immunoglobulin (in Guillain-Barre syndrome) and targeting cytokines in autoimmune disorders. A recent American Academy of Pain publication explains this new area of pain research further (2013).

Pain Genetics

In addition to the growing scientific evidence of psychological and environmental triggers for chronic pain, there is growing evidence of genetic factors. At the 15th World Congress on Pain in 2014, Mogil et al. presented evidence of "epigenetic changes" that signify permanent alterations in the transcription of certain genes affecting pain modulation that affect both pain sufferers *and their offspring* (2014). "The increase in pain sensitivity and psychological distress is thus facilitated through alteration of expression and activation of corresponding genes that code for biological pathways that represent potential drug targets," write the researchers. "Growing evidence suggests that chronic pain conditions are associated with both physical and psychological triggers, which initiate pain amplification and psychological distress; thus, susceptibility is dictated by complex interactions between genetic and environmental factors."

Every patient will develop such conditions via multiple pathways, say the researchers, governed by different probabilities defined by a complex interaction between the patient's genetic background and the extent of exposure to environmental events. As genes that code for biological pathways that represent potential drug targets continue to be discovered, we are gaining a better understanding of why certain drugs like morphine produce varied reactions in patients.

> Pain is increasingly being viewed as a set of probabilities defined by a complex interaction between the patient's genetic background and the extent of exposure to environmental events.

There are many existing and developing theories of pain which reveal how difficult it is to understand and treat. Burchiel says, "it is clear that pain perception is a highly complex phenomenon, and that there are no 'pain centers' in the brain that can be destroyed or removed" as can be done in some seizure disorders (2015).

Pain Theories at Work

We have learned so far that the experience we call "pain" is a complex process. The definition accepted by the International Association for the Study of Pain (IASP) is "Pain is an unpleasant sensory and emotional experience associated with actual or potential tissue damage, or described in terms of such damage." This is a good definition that has stood over time.

The pain process begins with nociception, the detection of noxious stimuli that are damaging to normal tissues by a soup of chemical mediators, as we see in Table 3.6. These messages are carried by a subset of primary neurons in the periphery by transduction, a process by which physical/mechanical, chemical and thermal stimuli evolve into electrical impulses. The impulses are then transmitted though a variety of ion-gated channels in nerves to the spinal cord and then to the brain where they are modulated by descending periphery chemical and neural mediators eventually reaching the brain where they are perceived.

The reaction of a patient is modified by genetic, immune, psychological, and epigenetic social, legal, and cultural factors. However, in any step along this linear process there is potential for "sensitization" in the periphery or in the CNS, leading to perception of persistent pain without a noxious event.

Many aspects of the popular pain theories can be observed when an actual nociceptive injury occurs. Imagine something heavy like a messenger bag or old-fashioned landline telephone drops on a patient's big toe. According to the Door Bell Theory, thermal, mechanical, or chemical mediators, activated by the event, are "transduced," modulated and transmitted to the brain, where they are perceived as pain and tell the patient that there is "visitor" at the door. Indeed, the nociceptive event occurred at the toe, which was injured and where the "visitor" is.

When the patient grabs his toe and rubs it, as most people instinctively do, it demonstrates evidence for the Gate Theory's "modulation" since the slow moving C-fiber nerve signals from rubbing the injury unseat the sharper and much faster moving pain signals from A-fibers, at least partially closing the gate and thus decreasing pain.

If the patient swears when the accident occurs, that is no surprise. There is increasing evidence that four-letter words also can alleviate pain, especially among people who do not normally curse. Scientists from Keele University found volunteers were able to keep their hands submerged in icy water for a longer time when they swore, whereas non-swear words did not extend their submerge time. A volley of foul words "taps into emotional brain" centers, said the researchers, accelerating heart rate, fight or flight and reducing pain (2011). These reactions appear to arise

Table 3.6 Pain process	
	Nociception
	Transduction
	Transmission
	Modulation
	Perception

in the right brain, whereas most language production occurs in the left cerebral hemisphere of the brain, said the researchers.

As the pain from the dropped messenger bag or telephone radiates, the brain will readily perceive both the *fact* of the pain and its causality, a self-injury which are conflicting perceptions under the Mismatch Theory. The patient's sensory-discriminative, affective-motivational and evaluative-cognitive dimensions, as described in the Neuromatrix Theory, and the activity of his limbic system, as described by the Brain-Based Pain Modulation, will affect his pain perception as will his "pain genetics."

As the injury manifests, a cascade of prostaglandins, histamine, and other chemicals is released and converted into electrical signals, a process called *transduction or translation*, providing evidence for the Chemical Theory. Nerve fibers in the skin and elsewhere transmit pain signals to the brain as the sympathetic nervous system (SNS) releases dampening chemicals. The nociception also activates the hypothalamic-pituitary-adrenocortical axis which will secrete other chemicals including cortisone and cortisol. According to the Spinal Cord Mechanisms theory, microglia will be produced by the dorsal horn and cytokines and chemokines will be produced by the immune system according to the Neuroimmune Interactions Theory.

In 24 h, as A-delta fibers, responsible for the sharp, immediate pain secede to the slower-moving C-fibers which cause a duller, generalized aching, chances are the toe has turned "black and blue" and the foot is swollen and is warm, purplish, sweaty and throbbing. This is because the A-delta fibers have directed the SNS to alter circulation and perspiration patterns, send more blood to the foot (causing swelling) and relax blood vessels, which allows more fluid to leak out.

Within 3–5 days, the swelling, redness, and activity of the sympathetic nervous system decreases, as does the pain. Over a period of a few days to a few weeks, the patient will begin to use his foot gingerly, employing the Gate Theory as he tries to find positions that block the C-fibers as he walks. Since it is "just" a bruised toe, the patient will no doubt not complain or exhibit dramatic pain behaviors, commensurate with the Psychological Factors, Social Modeling, and Loeser Model theories of pain. He will not receive undue attention from his family or people in his social circles because this is not an injury which is considered severe in his culture (Table 3.7).

In Chap. 4, we will explain CBT and relaxation techniques that can be taught to patients. In Chap. 5, we will explore how systems of reimbursement are supporting chronic pain treatments that are not evidence-based and in Chap. 6, we will explore treatments that are highly effective in chronic pain patients.

Table 3.7 Main points of this chapter

Unlike nociceptive pain, chronic pain appears not to serve a biologically useful purpose
Physical pain theories postulate a pain generator, gate mechanisms, and roles of neurotransmitters
Psycho/socio pain theories postulate social modeling, pain behavior, and belief systems
Almost all pain theories demonstrate how complex the phenomenon of pain is
Newer theories of pain are developing that advance traditional theories

References

1611 King James Version of Jeremiah 15:18.

Bennett, D. L. H., McMahon, S. B., & Salter, M. W. (2014). In S. Raja, & C. Sommer (Eds.), Refresher Courses, PAIN 2014: 15th World Congress on Pain. Washington, DC: International Association for the Study of Pain Press.

Burchiel, K. (Ed.). *Surgical management of pain* (p. 525). New York: Thieme.

Coghill, R. C., McHaffie, J. G., & Yen, Y. F. (2003). Neural correlates of interindividual differences in the subjective experience of pain. *Proceedings of the National Academy of Sciences, 100*, 8538–8542.

Dawes, J. M., Calvo, M., Perkins, J. R., Paterson, K., Kiesewetter, H., Hobbs, C., et al. (2011). CXCL5 mediates UVB irradiation-induced pain. *Science Translational Medicine, 3*, 90.

Deer, T. R., Leong, M. S., Buvanendran, A., Gordin, V., Kim, P. S., Panchal, S. J., et al. (Eds.). (2013). *Comprehensive treatment of chronic pain by medical, interventional, and integrative approaches*. Chicago: The American Academy of Pain Medicine.

Fink, R. (1997, September 23). Repetitive strain injury—The ghost that haunts 200 Front St. 2. *Fink and Associates Workers' Compensation Newsletter.*

Fishman, S., & Berger, L. (2001). *The war on pain.* New York: Harper Perennial.

Frieden, J. (2011, March 28). AAPM: State of mind can turn acute pain to chronic pain. *MedPage Today.*

Goodman, J. E., & McGrath, P. J. (2003). Mothers' modeling influences children's pain during a cold pressor task. *Pain, 104*(3), 559–565.

Henry, D. (2011). Central nervous system reorganization in a variety of chronic pain states: A review. *PM&R, 3*(12), 1116–1125.

Koyama, T., McHaffie, J. G., Laurienti, P. J., & Coghill, R. C. (2005). The subjective experience of pain: Where expectations become reality. *Proceedings of the National Academy of Sciences, 102*, 12950–12955.

Melzack, R. (1999). From the gate to the neuromatrix. *Pain, Suppl 6*, 121–126.

Melzack, R., & Wall, D. (1982). *The challenge of pain* (pp. 4–16). New York: Penguin.

Mogil, J. S., Diatchenko, L., & Fillingim, R. B. (2014). An Introduction to pain genetics. In S. Raja, & C. Sommer (Eds.), Pain 2014 Refresher Courses: 15th World Congress on Pain. Washington, DC: International Association for the Study of Pain Press.

Moseley, G. L. (2003). A pain neuromatrix approach to patients with chronic pain. *Manual Therapy 8*(3), 130–140. Retrieved from http://www.ncbi.nlm.nih.gov/pubmed/12909433

Ossipov, M. H., & Porreca, F. (2014). Central mechanisms of pain. In S. N. Raja, & C. L. Sommer (Eds.), PAIN 2014 Refresher Courses: 15th World Congress on Pain. Washington, DC: International Association for the Study of Pain Press.

Sayyahfar, S., Chavoshzadeh, Z., Khaledi, M., Madadi, F., Yeganeh, M. H., Sawamura, D., et al. (2013). Congenital insensitivity to pain with anhidrosis presenting with palmoplantar keratoderma. *Pediatric Dermatology, 30*(6), 754–756.

Tennant, F. (2014). Glial cell activation and neuroinflammation: How they cause centralized pain. *Practical Pain Management, 14*, 5.

Vince, G. (2005, November 2). Ease pain by taking a good look at yourself. *New Scientist.*

Visser, E. J., & Davies, S. (2010). *Pain Practice, 10*(2), 163.

Chapter 4
Cognitive Behavioral Coping Strategies

Kelly Smerz and Brad K. Grunert

Psychological factors play a major role in perception, reaction, and perpetuation of pain, especially in patients with chronic pain, as we have discussed in Chaps. 1, 2, and 3. From the inception of multidisciplinary pain programs, psychological approaches have been the most important component to change and reverse "pain behaviors" and for teaching patients new strategies and approaches to improve their function despite pain. These techniques have included a very strict "operant model" in which physicians/clinicians, family members, third party payers, and society in general do not reinforce pain behaviors but help the patient to unlearn pain and disability behavior and replace them with well and healthy behaviors.

Cognitive and Cognitive Behavioral treatments, which teach coping with pain while improving function, have been the most common psychological approach to chronic pain along with specific relaxation and breathing techniques and biofeedback. All are useful in teaching our patients living with chronic pain to decrease their pain perception and regain control over pain. That is why Howard Rusk, M.D., one of the leaders in the field of rehabilitation once said "Medicine has added years to life, but rehabilitation adds life to years."

This chapter, by Dr. Brad Grunert, a rehabilitation health psychologist and his colleague, Dr. Kelly Smerz, provides an excellent and up-to-date review of the role of the psychologist and Cognitive Behavioral coping strategies in helping patients with chronic pain. the evidence-based strategies. In conjunction with education,

K. Smerz, PhD
Milwaukee, WI, USA

B.K. Grunert, PhD
Department of Psychiatry and Behavioral Medicine, Medical College of Wisconsin, Milwaukee, WI, USA

Department of Plastic Surgery, Medical College of Wisconsin, Milwaukee, WI, USA

© Springer International Publishing Switzerland 2015
S. Vasudevan, *Multidisciplinary Management of Chronic Pain*,
DOI 10.1007/978-3-319-20322-5_4

appropriate medications and physical rehabilitation are essential components of a multidisciplinary approach to treating individuals with chronic pain.

Dr. Grunert is a trusted colleague with whom I have worked for the past 30 years and I extend my sincere gratitude to him and Dr. Smerz for their contribution to this book.

Sridhar Vasudevan, M.D.

Cognitive Behavioral Therapy (CBT) interventions are the most widely used psychological approaches to managing chronic pain. These approaches rely on several common elements. The first of these is providing a rationale for the intervention. The patient and therapist collaboratively define what chronic pain is, how it differs from acute pain, and the differences between managing acute versus chronic pain. The rationale for implementing each CBT intervention is then developed with the patient. It is essential that patients not only comprehend the nature of the intervention but that they also are active participants in developing a plan for implementation. This collaborative approach between the therapist and the patient provides a platform for modifying and customizing each intervention to the particular needs and demands of each patient's unique situation. While there are many similarities between patients in their development of a CBT intervention plan, the need for individualizing the plan is paramount to long-term success and commitment to managing chronic pain.

One of the frequent commonalities observed in the chronic pain population is the proclivity of patients to catastrophize their pain. Rather than developing strategies for coping with their pain, they engage in efforts to avoid provoking their pain. Typically this leads to decreasing activity, social withdrawal, and worsening depression. Patients begin to avoid the very things in their lives which made them meaningful simply as a means of controlling their exposure to pain. As this trend progresses, patients actually become physically debilitated, often to the point where they can no longer engage in previously enjoyable activities. They can no longer tolerate being up and around in social settings and their range of rewarding life experiences shrinks further. The loss of physical activity and social interaction results in depression and further isolation. By developing an understanding of the differences between acute and chronic pain, patients can formulate strategies to reverse these losses. Knowing that their chronic pain is benign and that decreasing activity and socialization will only magnify the morbidity associated with these conditions allows the chronic pain patient to consider alternate responses to their pain. This in turn assists them in abandoning the interventional role of medicine in "curing" their pain and leads to greater self-reliance in their pain management. It is at this point that CBT interventions are most likely to be successfully implemented into the management plan of the patient.

In this chapter we will present a variety of coping strategies for chronic pain. These will include: (1) relaxation/arousal reduction techniques; (2) self-talk; (3) stress-inoculation training; (4) internal distraction; (5) external distraction; (6) pacing; (7) mindfulness; and (8) acceptance and commitment strategies. While we will present basic components of each of these coping strategies, it is important to realize that these will only be successfully incorporated by the patient if they are personalized through collaboration with the individual who will be applying them. This collaborative process of tailoring the techniques is the core of the CBT intervention.

Relaxation/Arousal Reduction Techniques

Research shows that decreased arousal levels lead to a decreased subjective experience of pain and discomfort. There are a variety of techniques that have been developed to assist individuals in reducing their overall arousal level and consequently their subjective experience of pain. Relaxation training tends to enhance control over the individuals' arousal level. It also enhances a sense of personal control and self-efficacy for the individual practicing it. Pain tends to be magnified by anxiety and relaxation is an excellent means to counteract anxiety.

One of the primary techniques developed in order to achieve relaxation is autogenic relaxation (Jacobson 1962). With implementation of autogenic relaxation techniques, the individuals focus on a particular area of their body and devote their attention to this. They focus on the desired sensations in that area of the body that they wish to achieve. An example of this may be something as simple as mentally repeating "my hands feel warm and heavy," which they focus on in an almost meditative type of state. Systematically the individual would go through their entire body using various phrases to enhance their relaxation. There is a strong focus on controlled breathing throughout this type of relaxation. In many respects it shares a great deal with hypnotic induction except that there is no therapist who is conducting this with them.

Progressive muscle relaxation is a second technique that has been developed to assist individuals in reducing their overall arousal level (Bernstein and Borkovec 1973). Progressive muscle relaxation relies on a tension–relaxation cycle implemented by the individual. Again, the focus is on separate areas of the body at the beginning. This protocol initially begins with 16 muscle groups that are addressed in a systematic manner. The individual will tense the muscle group and then rapidly release the tension, triggering a relaxation response. As the patient becomes more proficient with this technique, the muscle groups are combined thereby shortening the induction. The speed with which the individual can achieve a deeply relaxed state increases. Again, there is a focus during this on controlling breathing to assist in triggering a deeply relaxed state.

Breathing control is a widely used relaxation technique. Deep controlled breaths allow patients to again decrease their arousal level. By taking a deep breath, holding it and then slowly exhaling, the individual can trigger a significant decrease in their overall arousal level. One of the advantages of using controlled breathing is that this is a technique that can be used anywhere at any time. It is not obvious to others when this is being implemented, even when out in public. The focus is truly internal and on an individual simply modulating their own breathing. This again enhances their sense of personal control and self-efficacy and gives them a relaxation technique that they can use anywhere, anytime.

A final technique that has been used to teach relaxation is biofeedback training. This can take a variety of forms. Typically, the individual is focusing on some type of physiologic feedback that is being provided to them with the goal of monitoring one's overall arousal level. By decreasing their arousal level in various forms, such as increasing their hand temperature, decreasing their muscle activity or decreasing their heart rate, patients can learn how to achieve a more relaxed state. This training is then gradually generalized until the individual is able to accomplish this without the need of actually having the monitoring equipment present. Again, they are frequently able to achieve a deeply relaxed state which again counters the increases in pain that they may experience in various situations.

Self-Talk

Self-talk refers to that inner dialogue, or inner narrator, that exists inside each of us. This narrator provides a running commentary on our thoughts, emotions, interactions, and behaviors as we navigate through daily life. The nature of this inner dialogue is influenced by past and current life experiences that shape beliefs, attitudes, assumptions, and habits. The cognitive therapy component of CBT recognizes that the content of our thoughts can have significant consequences for our emotional state and our behavior. Often we become so habituated to our own style of thinking that we do not notice what it is that we are saying to ourselves. When all is well, this may not be a problem. However, during times of stress and distress these automatic thoughts can become overly negative and highly detrimental to our emotional well-being.

Certain patterns of self-talk, or problematic thinking, are common among chronic pain patients and are important targets for therapy. Catastrophic thinking, for example, is something we observe frequently in our work with pain patients. It is also well documented in the pain psychology literature (Caudill 2009; Ehde et al. 2014). In catastrophic thinking, worries, fears, and other anxieties become amplified in a manner that unnecessarily heightens distress and compromises coping. These catastrophic fears can be about the pain itself (e.g., "My pain is worse today and therefore it will never improve") or the ways in which pain is perceived as impacting various aspects of the patient's life (e.g., "I'll never be able to do anything worthwhile again"). Negative beliefs and assumptions about oneself can also emerge as the person struggles to deal with the challenges of chronic pain. Changes or losses in valued roles or identities—breadwinner, homemaker, primary parent—can contribute to an inner dialogue that focuses on feelings of failure, worthlessness, and lack of value. If the despair associated with these thoughts is severe enough, suicidal thinking can ensue.

Cognitive therapy offers several strategies for targeting this maladaptive self-talk. Generally one of the first goals of treatment is to teach patients how to recognize their own self-talk. This can be challenging given that our thoughts patterns may be so subtle, automatic, or habitual, that we do not actually realize what we are saying to ourselves ("It's just how I think, doc."). After teaching the patient how to take his or her thoughts off "auto-pilot," it can then be helpful to facilitate a sense of curiosity as to where certain maladaptive thoughts patterns originated. This type of intervention can guide patients in questioning their own attitudes, beliefs, and schemas, which may or may not be accurate in the context of chronic pain (e.g., "Where did you learn that you have less value as a person if you are unable to work?"). Through this line inquiry, patients can learn to challenge, reframe, and rethink unhelpful thought patterns that are compromising their well-being.

Stress Inoculation Training

Stress inoculation training was developed by Meichenbaum (1977) as an iterative process to assist people in confronting stressful situations. It has been adapted for use with chronic pain patients as a means of assisting them in planning ahead and coping with situations and then refining their coping skills and abilities. Stress inoculation training is heavily reliant on skill acquisition and implementation with subsequent reevaluation and fine tuning of the process. Once skills are acquired by the individual, a plan for using them in response to particular stimuli or situations is developed. The skills can be any of the many cognitive coping skills that are discussed in this chapter. These skills are then applied in response to the stimuli which provoke increases in pain or present particular challenges to individuals encountering them. These challenges can include both the emotional aspects, as well as the physiologic demands of confronting various situations. After the individual addresses the set of stressful stimuli and incorporates the coping plan, the application is then reviewed with identification of strengths and weaknesses of the implementation as it took place. This is then followed up by additional planning and skill acquisition for future implementation when this particular constellation of stressors is again encountered.

An example of applying stress inoculation training in the context of chronic pain may be something as simple as shopping at a mall. It is important to identify what the constraints of the situation are. The individual hopefully will have a map of the shopping mall available to them. They can then plan how far it is for them to ambulate from an area where they park into the mall. They can identify appropriate rest points where they can sit and practice some of the skills available to them. They can focus on whether or not they are able to pace themselves appropriately and build in stop points throughout the entire task. Additionally, they can identify whether or not they need a cart or someone to accompany them in order to carry any of the goods that they buy.

These patients also need to determine what skills are available to them and how applicable these are to the particular setting. These skills may include techniques such as internal distraction, appropriate self-talk, external distraction or pacing. They then proceed with implementing the plan. Following this they go back and revisit how successful they were in accomplishing the task that they outlined and how successful they were in implementing their skillset to cope with the difficulties that arose. This troubleshooting after the implementation is a key part of the entire stress inoculation training process. Following this, the individual then formulates a new plan for their next trip to the mall identifying some of the trouble spots and also strategies that they can utilize to overcome these.

Used in this manner, stress inoculation training is an ongoing process helping individuals to refine their skills and to develop new skills that they may need in order to cope with particular situations that arose and posed significant challenges for them. They can also develop a plan anticipating when they will experience an increase in pain during the entire process. This anticipation can then be planned for with implementation of an appropriate set of skills to assist them in managing their pain. This iterative process continues until the individuals feel capable and confident in confronting the situation that they have been exposed to while applying their pain management plan.

Internal Distraction

Guided imagery and hypnosis interventions can provide a source of internal distraction from chronic pain. These interventions generally focus not only on diminishing the experience of the pain itself, but also on enhancing well-being and empowerment and reducing emotional arousal and distress. Although generally taught in the clinician's office, both guided imagery and self-hypnosis are tools given to the patient to practice at home. In fact, at home practice is a strongly encouraged aspect of this treatment modality.

Belleruth Naparstek, who is well-known for her work in the area of guided imagery, describes this imagery process as "a kind of directed day dreaming" (1994, p. 4). She notes that in guided imagery, the power of the imagination is used to promote physical healing and emotional well-being. According to Naperstack, effective imagery interventions incorporate all of the senses and generally involve an altered state of awareness characterized by both a relaxed focus and energized alertness. Hypnosis is often described quite similarly, and Jensen and Patterson (2014) remark that it can be difficult to determine when an intervention crosses into a hypnotic realm. As such, there may be a fine line that exists between guided imagery and hypnosis.

Guided imagery and hypnotic interventions for chronic pain often incorporate images and suggestions for pain reduction and relaxation. Naparstek (1994) encourages the use of images that help the person "soften" and "open" to the experience of the pain. She explains that pain sensations are better managed when we learn to relax and breathe into them. This helps to counteract or natural inclination to resist and "wall-off," which can paradoxically heighten the pain. Images and suggestions for improvements in sleep, coping, energy, and mood—the attendant disruptions of chronic pain—also seem to be important. In fact, research has shown that use of hypnosis to improve these other associated symptoms of pain is important in patient satisfaction, even if the pain itself is only temporarily or minimally improved (Jensen and Patterson 2014).

External Distraction

External distraction strategies comprise another set of coping behaviors that are likely to benefit those with chronic pain. These strategies address important aspects of the social and emotional withdrawal that can turn physical pain into emotional suffering. Primary among these interventions are those that assist patients in rebuilding social relationships. This often means learning how to once again enjoy quality time and activities with friends, family, and important others. Patients may need guidance and training in learning to assert various needs arising from their pain condition. For example, they may need physical assistance, activity modification, or adjusted expectations. For patients who have historically been very self-reliant, asking a friend to drop them off at the door, or asking a partner to stay for one, rather than 3 h at a social gathering, can feel very shameful and anxiety inducing. It is therefore important for healthcare providers to concurrently work with patients on managing any self-talk that might undermine their ability to effectively assert their needs.

Research studies demonstrate the incredible importance of social relationships and social support. Loneliness, for example, has been shown to be a predictor of pain, depression, and fatigue symptoms in cancer survivors and in older adults caring for a spouse with dementia (Jaremka et al. 2014). Moreover, this same study found that loneliness not only predicted present symptoms, but also an increase in these symptoms over time. In another study, loneliness in fibromyalgia patients was related to heightened pain and greater perception of stress during interpersonal interactions. In this population, the impact of loneliness on quality of life persisted even after accounting for daily depression (Wolf and Davis 2014).

Hobbies and activities can provide other sources of external distraction. These can be instrumental in helping the patient structure his or her day. They can also provide a sense of meaning and purpose, which have been shown to be important to the well-being of patients with chronic health conditions (Dezutter et al. 2013). When identifying realistic hobbies and activities, creativity is key. Is there a way to adapt something that was enjoyed prepain condition so that it accommodates the patient's limitations? Alternately, patients can benefit from discussions that help them explore new activity options that perhaps were never considered in their busy, preinjury lives.

Pacing

Physical limitations are a frustration for many pain patients. Chores, work duties, hobbies, and activities once accomplished with ease suddenly become exhausting and pain inducing. As part of a broader repertoire of effective coping, many pain patients find benefit in learning to pace themselves. Pacing is based on the awareness that our physical energy and stamina are limited. Consequently, each and every day we all have to decide how we want to allocate these finite energies. The dilemma for pain patients is that these finite energies are usually markedly reduced from their preinjury functioning.

Pain patients often fall into one of two groups. The first group consists of those who are frustrated by their limitations and resist adjusting their activity level accordingly. These are the patients that can find themselves in a cycle in which they overdo it, are then disabled by pain for several days, and then overdo it again when the pain eases up. Comprising the second group are those who have significantly curtailed their activity as a consequence of their pain, thereby causing muscle deconditioning and an attendant loss of strength and stamina.

In the book *Managing Pain Before it Manages You*, Margaret Caudill (2009) suggests a series of pacing-related interventions that can be helpful to both groups. She suggests that patients can benefit from learning to listen to their bodies. This means not only knowing one's limits, but also recognizing when to alternate or change activities in service of preserving one's stamina. She also discusses the importance of *adaptation* and *delegating*. Adaptation involves finding new, innovative, and less pain inducing ways of accomplishing tasks. This can be applied not only to chores, but also to hobbies (e.g., sitting while cooking if standing is painful; using a higher desk or table for arts and craft projects is painful). Delegating involves "job sharing" and asking others for assistance.

For the group of deconditioned patients, pacing also involves learning to distinguish discomfort from pain (Turk and Winter 2006). Any activity, even if reasonable, can cause discomfort in weakened muscles. Education related to deconditioning, and discussions regarding reasonable stamina building activities and goals, can be important with this group. The collaboration of a physical therapist can also be helpful.

Teaching patients to manage anxious or maladaptive self-talk is also important to successful pacing interventions. Providers may need to work with patients on challenging "all or nothing thoughts," such as beliefs that if I cannot clean my house as meticulously as before I am somehow failing." Discussions and interventions may also need to address other maladaptive thought patterns such as those that make it unacceptable to ask for help, to delegate, or to adjust the expectations one maintains for him- or herself.

When Managing Cognitions and Behaviors Doesn't Manage the Pain

Although CBT has received widespread recognition by practitioners, researchers, and insurance companies as the "gold standard" of psychological interventions for chronic pain, there is an emerging body of research suggesting there may be more we can do. On the whole, Cognitive Behavioral interventions seem to be modestly to moderately effective in improving symptoms and disability (Ehde et al. 2014; Hoffman et al. 2007; Williams et al. 2012). However, concerns are beginning to emerge regarding some of the basic assumptions of CBT. Assertions regarding the importance, or even the necessity, of changing thought patterns and thought content in order to bring about more effective pain coping are being reconsidered in light of interventions that emphasize emotional awareness, tolerance, and acceptance (McCracken and Vowles 2014).

Turning Toward the Pain

The notion of psychologically turning toward one's pain is a concept that is at best foreign, and perhaps even quite aversive, for many pain patients. To imagine both looking at one's pain and learning to relate to it, is, for many, a veritable contradiction to life in a society that teaches us that we should not have to think uncomfortable thoughts, nor should we have to feel distressing emotions. Unwanted sensations, emotions, and experiences are things to be avoided, numbed, escaped, or quickly fixed. Unfortunately, for many pain patients, there are neither quick fixes nor easy answers, but instead, many frustrations and an abundance of coping challenges.

Mindfulness is an approach to psychotherapy that embraces the notion of turning toward the pain. Recognizing the paradox of chronic pain, it encourages patients to consider and explore the possibility that relief can be found by learning to relate to their pain, rather than running from it. Likewise, mindfulness addresses the manner in which attempts to dampen or avoid the awareness of pain can inadvertently worsen emotional and physical distress (Dahl and Lundgren 2006; Kabat-Zinn 2010 Disks One and Two; Siegel 2005). Efforts to avoid or manage thoughts, behaviors, and situations that might exacerbate pain, often result in viscous feedback loops of heightened anxiety and depression, catastrophic thinking, amplified pain, and behavioral restriction. This cycle can ultimately contribute to significant disability and distress, and a great deal of needless suffering.

Mindfulness approaches to the management of chronic pain differ from cognitive and Cognitive Behavioral interventions primarily in two ways (Jensen and Turk 2014). The first difference lies in how the respective approaches guide the patient in handling unwanted cognitions and distressing emotions. In other words, they differ in their approach to the question of "What to do about it." Traditional cognitive interventions emphasize the importance of the patient learning to recognize how certain cognitions, in the form of beliefs, attitudes, and self-talk, can contribute to unhelpful patterns and processes of thinking. These habitual, unhelpful, and "maladaptive" thought patterns become the target of therapeutic modification and restructuring, and patients are taught cognitive management strategies such as examining, challenging, reframing, and reconsidering. By contrast, with mindfulness interventions, patients learn to relate differently to their thoughts. Thoughts, and their attendant emotions, are not seen as something that should, or even can, be controlled. Instead, relief is found through mindfulness techniques that teach the patient how to become less identified with the thoughts, which are seen as merely products of the mind that have a life of their own (Eifert and Forsyth 2005; Kabat-Zinn 2010, Disks One and Two).

The second difference between the approaches lies in the question of how to bring about well-being. In cognitive therapy, the goal is to learn how to engage productively with one's thoughts in service of enhancing feelings of empowerment and a sense of control. Cognitive theory asserts that uncomfortable emotions diminish when the thoughts that drive them are no longer functioning like a runaway train. Mindfulness, on the other hand, has the goal of diminishing engagement with one's thoughts in service of disentangling from unproductive efforts to control what cannot be controlled. When patients are no longer trying to suppress, control, or fix their thoughts or emotions, the result is a reduction in emotional reactivity and greater freedom to connect with inherent possibilities for living that exist in the present moment (Kabat-Zinn 2010).

These differences between CBT and mindfulness were demonstrated in a studying that examined the respective benefits of these therapies in a group of rheumatoid arthritis patients (Zautra et al. 2008). What the authors found was that the Cognitive Behavioral intervention was associated with improvements in cognitive control of pain, and the mindfulness intervention resulted in better emotion regulation. The authors also found that the mindfulness intervention was particularly effective for patients with recurrent depression. When compared to CBT and an education-only control group, those with recurrent depression who received the mindfulness intervention experienced greater enhancement of positive affect, greater reduction in negative affect and a greater reduction in pain as measured by physician-assessed joint swelling and tenderness. The authors conclude that the manner in which the mindfulness intervention connected the patients with positive emotional and social resources may have been especially beneficial for those with depression.

In the therapeutic context, mindfulness is often taught in the form of meditational type exercises that cultivate both centering and awareness. As an example, patients can be taught to focus on their breath, to notice when they become distracted and what distracted them, and to return their focus to their breath, doing this over and over again during the course of any meditation (Germer 2005; Kabat-Zinn 2010, Disk Two). As patients learn to notice their mental distractions without reacting to them, they learn about the inner workings of their mind.

Regardless of how it is taught, mindfulness is about learning to be present, fully and nonjudgmentally, in the moments unfolding of our lives. Mindful is often confused with relaxation strategies when it is first introduced in therapy. It is therefore important to explain to patients that this is neither the goal, nor will it be attainable on all occasions (Eifert and Forsyth 2005; Kabat-Zinn 2005; Siegel 2005). Rather, meditation is about learning to remain psychologically present with the moment-to-moment awareness of one's thoughts, feelings, and sensations—one's internal experiences. Mindfulness also involves cultivating a nonjudgmental attitude toward whatever arises in the awareness (Kabat-Zinn 2005). For those with chronic pain, this means learning to stay present with whatever pain-related thoughts, feelings, and sensations arise without judging, evaluating, or trying to change what is.

As patients learn to be, and stay, present with what goes on internally, they become less fearful of their inner experience and less inclined toward psychological escape. Emotional reactivity diminishes as patients feel increasingly safe with their cognitions and emotions (Germer 2005), and opportunities to develop new ways of relating to the pain emerge. Ultimately, patients develop compassion for themselves, they learn how to respond mindfully rather than reactively, and they develop a sense of self that extends beyond the pain (Kabat-Zinn 2010, CDs One and Two). Although it can also be taught informally in form of mindful awareness, it has been suggested that "Mindfulness has to be experienced to be known" (Germer 2005). Support for taking a more formal approach also comes from research suggesting that the regular practice of mindfulness meditation reduces pain sensitivity (Grant et al. 2010).

Acceptance and Commitment Therapy

Acceptance and Commitment Therapy (ACT) is another psychological approach that addresses the coping challenges encountered by chronic pain patients. The ACT model of treatment extends CBT and blends it with some of the basic principles of mindfulness such as acceptance and emotional tolerance (McCracken and Vowles 2014). Like many other psychological interventions for chronic pain, ACT addresses the role of fear and experiential avoidance in the maintenance of both the emotional sequelae and physical symptoms of chronic pain. Where ACT diverges from more traditional Cognitive Behavioral interventions is in its focus on reducing emotional suffering rather than reducing pain, per se. Fundamental to ACT is the belief that suffering diminishes when individuals learn a different way of relating to their pain—a way that is open, flexible, and life affirming.

Psychological flexibility is one of the fundamental and overarching tenets of ACT (McCracken and Vowles 2014). In the context of ACT, psychological flexibility can be thought of as the ability to effectively adapt one's behavior, as guided by one's values, to accommodate the ever changing intrapsychic and external demands of a situation. Also important to this definition is the notion that these behavioral adaptations allow for greater and more meaningful contact with the present in service of living a valued life. In the context of chronic pain, psychological flexibility can help an individual avoid becoming stuck in the rigid, entrenched, and maladaptive coping styles that can arise from beliefs and rules about the pain and how one should cope.

Also fundamental to ACT is the notion that experiential avoidance is central to the exacerbation and maintenance of symptoms (Dahl et al. 2005; Eifert and Forsyth 2005; Hayes 2004). Experiential avoidance can be thought of as the efforts one exerts to control and avoid distressing internal experiences (i.e., thoughts, emotions, memories, bodily sensations). What ACT recognizes is that there is often a paradoxical effect to efforts to avoid and control these internal awarenesses. Trying not to think about pain, or anxiety, or depression for that matter, actually activates that thought, "I am in pain (or anxious or depressed)," and leaves the patient unintentionally more entangled and distressed by the thing he hoped to control and avoid. These types of efforts often result in what Dahl and Lundgren (2006) have called "dirty pain," which is pain complicated by frustrations, self-directed admonitions, distressing emotions, and unproductive efforts to avoid and control one's experience. Dirty pain is the type of pain that can turn physical pain into emotional suffering.

As a therapy, ACT is particularly relevant to the treatment needs of chronic pain patients. Although there is no set protocol for ACT, most therapies address the topics of cognitive defusion, mindfulness and self as context, acceptance, values identification, and committed action. (See Dahl and Lundgren 2006 for an excellent example of a treatment protocol.) Each of these concepts will be described below.

Cognitive defusion is an important intervention that addresses the tendency of our human mind to confuse our thoughts about something with the thing itself (Dahl et al. 2005; Eifert and Forsyth 2005; Hayes 2004). This cognitive "confusion" is known as *cognitive fusion*. As an example, we can take a look at a common belief among individuals dealing with chronic pain. The line of thinking goes—"*I am in pain; my body is damaged; therefore I am damaged.*" This logic pattern then extends and activates other thoughts, feelings, beliefs, and rules about the value of damaged people (e.g., less worthy) and what damaged people can and cannot, and should and should not do (e.g., should not reach out to others because they will be a burden). What becomes readily apparent in this example is how the awareness of one's pain becomes fused with beliefs that diminish one's self-esteem and create social isolation. Cognitive defusion interventions help the person gain distance from their thoughts by looking *at* one's thoughts rather than *from* one's thoughts (Hayes 2004). This works toward disentangling one's identity, behavior, and lifestyle decisions from the pain.

Mindfulness and Self as Context: As discussed earlier in this chapter, mindfulness is a tool that cultivates the capacity to tolerate, and be less reactive to, unwanted thoughts, feelings, and sensations. When offered within the framework of ACT, mindfulness becomes a tool for practicing cognitive defusion. It is also instrumental in learning to tolerate distressing internal experiences. Through the practice of mindfulness, patients learn to recognize mental processes as cognitive events, not literal truths (Hayes 2004). ACT-based mindfulness exercises also work toward the internal cultivation of an observer, or transcendent, self that is constant, steady and more than the experience that is happening at the moment (Dahl and Lundgren 2006; Dahl et al. 2005; Hayes 2004). This notion of self as context is often taught in the form of an exercise that demonstrates how "you have been you your whole life" despite constantly changing circumstances and emotions. For pain patients this awareness means that *you are more than your pain*.

Acceptance: The notion of acceptance is also integral to ACT. In the context of this therapy, acceptance is not a passive surrendering, nor is it a form of giving up (Eifert and Forsyth 2005). It is an active engagement with life that involves "living with what you cannot control, even if it's unpleasant, *and* actively pursuing the life you want" (Dahl and Lundgren 2006, p. 112). Acceptance requires cognitive defusion and mindfulness, which together encourages the patient to experience the moment as it is, not something to be evaluated, judged, or changed. As Hayes (2004, p. 656) writes, "This means feeling feelings as feelings, thinking thoughts as thoughts, sensing sensations as sensations, and so on, here and now."

Jensen, M. P., & Turk, D. C. (2014). Contributions of psychology to the understanding and treatment of people with chronic pain: Why it matters to all psychologists. *American Psychologist, 69*(2), 105–118.

Kabat-Zinn, J. (2005). *Wherever you go there you are*. New York: Hyperion.

Kabat-Zinn, J. (2010). *Mindfulness meditation for pain relief*. Session One [Audio CD]. Boulder, CO: Sounds True.

McCracken, L. M., Gutierrez-Martinez, O., & Smyth, C. (2013). "Decentering" reflects psychological flexibility in people with chronic pain and correlates with their quality of functioning. *Health Psychology, 32*(7), 820–823.

McCracken, L. M., & Vowles, K. E. (2014). Acceptance and commitment therapy and mindfulness for chronic pain: Model, Process, and Progress. *American Psychologist, 69*(2), 178–187.

Meichenbaum, D. H. (1977). *Cognitive-behavior modification: An integrative approach*. New York: Plenum.

Naparstek, B. (1994). *Staying well with guided imagery*. New York: Warner Books.

Ruiz, F. (2010). A review of acceptance and commitment therapy (ACT) empirical evidence: Correlational, experimental, psychopathology, component, and outcome studies. *International Journal of Psychology and Psychological Therapy, 10*(1), 125–162.

Siegel, R. D. (2005). Psychophysiological disorders: Embracing pain. In C. K. Germer, R. D. Siegel, & P. R. Fulton (Eds.), *Mindfulness and psychotherapy* (pp. 173–196). New York: The Guilford Press.

Turk, D. C., & Winter, F. (2006). *The pain survival guide: How to reclaim your life*. Washington, DC: American Psychological Association.

Vowles, K. E., & McCracken, L. M. (2008). Acceptance and values-based action in chronic pain: A study of treatment effectiveness and process. *Journal of Consulting and Clinical Psychology, 76*(3), 397–407.

Wicksell, R. K., Ahlqvist, J., Bring, A., Melin, L., & Olsson, G. L. (2008). Can exposure and acceptance strategies improve functioning and quality of life in people with chronic pain and whiplash associated disorders (WAD)? A randomized control trial. *Cognitive Behaviour Therapy, 37*(3), 1–14.

Williams, A. C., Eccleston, C., & Morley, S. (2012). Psychological therapies for the management of chronic pain (excluding headache) in adults. *Cochrane Database of Systematic Reviews, 11*, CD007407.

Wolf, L. D., & Davis, M. C. (2014). Loneliness, daily pain, and perceptions of interpersonal events in adults with fibromyalgia. *Health Psychology, 33*(9), 929–937.

Zautra, A. J., Davis, M. C., Reich, J. W., Nicassario, P., Tennen, H., Finan, P., et al. (2008). Comparison of cognitive behavioral and mindfulness meditation interventions on adaptation to rheumatoid arthritis for patients with and without history of recurrent depression. *Journal of Consulting and Clinical Psychology, 76*(3), 408–421.

Chapter 5
Treatments That Have Questionable or Controversial Evidence

Note about this chapter:

This chapter does not address the treatment of patients with acute and subacute pain. It does not address patients with a herniated disk with nerve compression and radiculopathy (pain down a nerve distribution in the arms below the elbow and in the legs below the knee) who, on the basis of objective neurological findings of these conditions can benefit from an epidural injection and/or discectomy, if properly selected and motivated. Nor does this chapter address patients with pain from malignant sources, patients receiving appropriate physical or chiropractic therapy who may require opioids to increase participation in their treatment/rehabilitation process or patients who require surgical treatment for traumatic fracture of the limbs or spine to stabilize the fracture towards healing.

*What this chapter **does** address is the use of surgery, injections, other interventions and chronic opioid therapy for patients with chronic pain as we have described and defined it in earlier chapters. For these patients there is questionable evidence despite their widespread use.*

If one fact unifies all the advances in chronic nonmalignant pain research in the last 40 years, it is that pain is complex. There is rarely a single cause or treatment much as we and our patients would wish.

For years, pain was viewed through a simplistic theory of peripheral nociception initiating a neural impulse transmitted to the brain. However, we now know pain is modulated not just in the peripheral but in the central nervous system. The Gate Theory of pain (Melzack and Wall 1988), discussed in Chap. 2, led to the intense study of the dorsal horn of the spinal cord in neuromodulation. We know now that neurotransmitters like substance P, norepinephrine, serotonin, GABA, and endorphins are involved in pain, providing us a mechanistic approach in using pharmacological and physical agents to relieve pain.

© Springer International Publishing Switzerland 2015
S. Vasudevan, *Multidisciplinary Management of Chronic Pain*,
DOI 10.1007/978-3-319-20322-5_5

Table 5.1 Common pain interventions in patients with chronic pain

Treatment	Short-term relief	Long-term relief	Costly	Need to be repeated
Surgeries	Maybe	Maybe	Yes	Maybe
Injections/blocks	Yes	No	Yes	Yes
Spine stimulators	Yes	Maybe	Yes	No
Denervation/ ablation	Yes	Maybe	Yes	Maybe
Opioids	Yes	No	No	Yes
Multidisciplinary pain rehabilitation	Maybe	Yes	Maybe	No

Medical professionals treating pain also know now that a patient's pain experience is greatly affected by social, familial, cultural, vocational, and financial factors as well as emotional states like depression, anger, fear, anxiety, and feelings of powerlessness and victimization.

Sadly, even as we appreciate chronic pain's complexity and the validity of the Biopsychosocial model, treatments are reverting to a single-cause biological model thanks to the way health care is delivered and reimbursed. Contemporary chronic pain treatment, especially in the United States, is characterized by expensive, often uncoordinated treatments that produce poor outcomes and often lack evidence base as shown in Table 5.1. This system has largely phased out multidisciplinary care for chronic pain which is incorrectly viewed as more costly than unimodal treatments despite superior long-term outcomes in pain, disability, return to work, reduction in narcotic use, and repeat hospitalizations and surgery (Meier 2013). Ironically, in countries other than the United States, multidisciplinary pain treatment is expanding.

In 2014, the Obama administration announced that it will begin "coordinating" some Medicare services, an admission of how uncoordinated care has become. While physicians have often coordinated and managed care for their patients without being compensated, they will now be paid "to coordinate the care of Medicare beneficiaries, amid growing evidence that patients with chronic illnesses suffer from disjointed, fragmented care," according to an administration announcement (Pear 2014). Officials said such coordination of care could "pay for itself by keeping patients healthier and out of hospitals."

One indication of the extent to which non-EBM (Evidence-Based Medicine) treatments for chronic pain and the uncoordinated care in which they flourish have become established is the phenomenon of "failed back surgery syndrome" or FBSS. The term applies to an estimated 10–40 % of patients who receive only modest improvement after back surgery or none at all (Lee and Vasudevan 2012). FBSS is an umbrella term that does not specify the patient's prior diagnosis, the reason for surgery failure or any present symptoms. Several studies list spinal stenosis, disk disruption or retained disk and epidural fibrosis as the most common causes of FBSS followed by recurrent disk herniations, iatrogenic instability, facet pain, and sacroiliac joint pain.

Yet despite the growth of FBSS in the United States, it is an ailment that "does not exist in most of the world," writes Peter Abaci in *Take Charge of Your Chronic Pain* (2010) because "Most other countries don't perform spine surgeries at the high rate that we do in the United States." Comparable conditions like "failed hip surgery syndrome" or "failed knee surgery syndrome" don't exist. The rate of back surgery in the United States is five times that in the United Kingdom according to the American Pain Society's Guideline for the Evaluation and Management of Low Back Pain Evidence Review (2007). It is reported to be double that of Australia, Canada, and Finland (Lee and Vasudevan 2012).

The pendulum has swung back to the time when there was little awareness that a patient's experience of pain was affected by his mental and emotional state, family and finances, and legal and vocational factors. While treatments like spinal fusions and disk surgery, spinal cord stimulators, steroid and painkiller injections, nerve ablation and of course long-term prescription of narcotics have greatly increased in the United States in the last decade, so has the incidence of adults who report chronic pain, which has actually doubled (Wells-Federman 1999; IOM 2011). Clearly, the newer methods are not working.

Dr. John Loeser, Professor Emeritus of neurological surgery, anesthesiology and pain medicine at the University of Washington who developed the Loeser Model of pain reviewed in Chap. 3, has also noted that the "purely medical" approach that dominates current chronic pain treatment, disregards "psychological and social factors" (IASP 2013). *Others are also addressing the US's drift away from treating the person in preference for treating the "pain" with expensive but often ineffective treatments.*

"We don't use our expensive drugs and technologies appropriately. Instead of using these interventions to benefit patients, we use them to maximize revenues, and often harm patients," writes Otis Webb Brawly, M.D., chief medical officer of the American Cancer Society and author of *How We Do Harm* (Brawley 2011). As it stands, says Dr. Brawley, "abominable" care is often the rule not the exception because "the patient knows the science but chooses to ignore it," physicians often gravitate to the most expensive care and "the insurance company has no access to adequate information."

An especially controversial area in chronic pain care is surgical treatment of back pain. Lower back pain (LPB) is the second most frequent reason to visit a physician for a chronic condition, the fifth most common cause of hospitalization, and the third most frequent reason for a surgical procedure (Wheeler et al. 2013). It is the most common cause of disability in Americans younger than 45. In fact, LBP is so prevalent, the patient *without* it is actually more rare than the patient who has it.

Many back surgeries have shockingly low success rates. Second operations on the lumbar spine caused by new or recurrent pain, device failures and complications following the first operation are remarkably common and second and subsequent operations on lumbar spine are even less likely to be successful (Deyo and Mirza 2009). "One study on the Workers' Compensation population found that the success rate after a second lumbar surgical procedure was only 53 %, after a third operation it was 35 % and after a fourth or fifth operation it was reported being worse than being improved," reports a study in *European Spine Journal*.

"Even if the back surgery is successful in relieving pain, it can cause other problems," says Dr. Abaci (Abaci 2010). "People who have had spine surgery age differently over time. The support structures of their spines seem to wear out quicker in the areas where they had the surgery, leading to advanced degeneration of the disks and joints needed to support the back."

Nor is spine surgery the only procedure getting a second look. In 2014, a study, published in *Arthritis & Rheumatology* found that more than a third of total knee replacements performed in the United States were "inappropriate."

Spinal Fusion

Some time ago, a complex operation called spinal fusion in which metal rods are screwed into the spine to stabilize it emerged as the treatment of choice for many kinds of back pain. Yet researchers questioned and continue to question whether spinal fusions are preferable to lower cost laminectomies, from which patients recover more quickly or preferable to having no surgery at all as shown in Table 5.2 (Abelson and Petersen 2003).

An article in the *European Spine Journal* (Deyo and Mirza 2009) finds a dramatic increase in fusion rates after 1996 when intervertebral interbody fusion cage hardware used to hold two vertebrae apart while the fusion becomes solid were introduced, correlating with a 100 % increase in spine fusions paid by Medicare. "During the last 5 years of the 1990s, spine surgery rates in the Medicare population increased 40 %; spine fusion rates increased 70 %; and instrumented spinal fusions increased 100 %," write the authors. Some physicians suggested that fewer than half of fusions were appropriate and the expensive hardware employed could be driving the procedures' popularity.

In a presidential address for the Scoliosis Research Society, orthopedic surgeon Harry Shufflebarger cited a "fusion cage explosion," and stated that "the efficacy of these stand-alone devices is very questionable" after 4 years of use (Deyo and Mirza 2009). Patients with fusion instrumentation have a substantially higher likelihood of repeat surgery, higher rates of nerve injury, greater blood loss, longer operative time, and a higher rate of overall complications than seen with "decompression

Table 5.2 Limitations of spinal fusion surgery

Drawback	Details
Highly expensive surgery	4×cost of discectomy or laminectomy
A year required for recovery	Other surgeries require only weeks
May be overused; not always appropriate	Financial incentives/marketing to surgeons
Complications in 20 % of patients	Screws break loose, grafts/cages migrate
High rate of repeat surgeries	Fusion breakdown; other repairs

alone" write the authors. Early complications following fusion occur in up to 20 % of patients, say American Pain Society guidelines (2007) and the rate of in- hospital mortality is <1 %.

Many patients "who have had one fusion surgery require at least one more back operation at some point in their lives, often because the areas above and below the fusion break down and need repair," says Dr. Abaci (Abaci 2010).

The debate over the appropriateness of spinal fusions has spilled over from the pain field into general discussion of health care policy and allocation of resources. In *How Doctors Think*, Jerome Groopman, M.D. (2007) Professor of Medicine at Harvard Medical School and Chief of Experimental Medicine at Beth Israel Deaconess Medical Center observes that "the financial incentive tips heavily toward fusion" because the hardware generates "high profits" for the manufacturers and "the hospitals that use them" (Groopman 2007). At one hospital, for example, the surgeon's full fee for a simple discectomy is around $5000, writes Dr. Groopman, while compensation for a fusion surgery is $20,000. "For the majority of patients with chronic lumbar pain, fusion surgery has no dramatic impact on either their pain or their mobility. Yet many surgeons pay scant attention to the poor results," charges Dr. Groopman.

Nortin Hadler, Attending Rheumatologist at the University of North Carolina Hospitals and a graduate of Yale College and Harvard Medical School, concurs. "There is not a hint that surgery for regional back pain is helpful. There is barely a hint that surgery for radicular pain might be helpful," he writes in *Worried Sick* (Hadler 2008). In *Stabbed in the Back: Confronting Back Pain in an Overtreated Society*, Dr. Hadler disputes whether low back pain is an "injury" at all and traces its historical roots as a patient complaint and a medical diagnosis.

Dr. Hadler reserves particular criticism for what he calls a lucrative franchise built around back injuries in the Workers' Compensation system, noting the United States is the "first in the 'advanced' world" in surgically treating "the lumbosacral spines of workers."

"These claimants are victims of social iatrogenesis [physician-caused maladies]…seduced into thinking that their regional low back pain is a disabling injury consequent to a workplace accident. They are forced to use the painfulness to validate their request for indemnified health care." There is something profoundly wrong with a system that forces a patient to exhibit pain behaviors, continues Dr. Hadler. "If you have to prove you are ill, you can't get well." (Chapter 7 addresses disability and worker-related insurance systems in depth.)

Driving the popularity of fusions are companies like Medtronic, one of the biggest makers of spinal hardware, originally based in Minneapolis but seeking to reincorporate in Ireland in 2014. A lawsuit filed against Medtronic in 2001 and settled, accused the company of offering surgeons first-class plane tickets to Hawaii, nights at the finest hotels, consulting contracts that involved no work and outright kickbacks for their spinal hardware business (Abelson and Petersen 2003).

In affidavits provided to the press, about 80 surgeons were shown to have consulting agreements with Medtronic that paid as much as $400,000 a year and sales representatives even took surgeon prospects to strip clubs. At the University of Wisconsin in Madison, Thomas Zdeblick, M.D., chairman of the medical school's orthopedic department and a prominent spine surgeon received more than $25 million from Medtronic between 2003 and 2011 and the university hospital spent $27 million for Medtronic spinal products from 2004 to 2010 (Fauber 2011). The hospital equipped 179 patients with Medtronic devices between 2008 and 2011. Clearly, financial incentives can drive the choice of one surgery over another.

When the US Agency for Health Care Policy and Research attempted to establish back surgery guidelines that recommended a conservative approach and discouraged surgery, Medtronic successfully sued to have the recommendations kept from the public. The North American Spine Society, the main professional group for back surgeons, "launched an assault on the methods used by the AHCPR experts, charging that the agency had wasted taxpayer dollars on the study" according to press reports and almost succeeded in eliminating its funding (Brownlee 2007).

Medtronic has also been in the news over Infuse, its aggressively marketed bone graft material used in spine surgeries. An article in the *Bone & Joint Journal* by paid Medtronic consultant, Timothy R. Kuklo, a former surgeon at Walter Reed Army Medical Center, was retracted (Wilson and Meier 2009) due to falsified data. According to an Army investigation, Dr. Kuklo reported much higher success rates in healing the shattered legs of wounded soldiers than was accurate.

"During his time at Walter Reed, Dr. Kuklo was extensively involved in research and writing about various Medtronic products, including editing two books published by the company [Medtronic] and conducting three studies that were approved by his Army superiors, according to his list of publications and an Army report," reported the *New York Times*.

In 2008, Infuse received a Food and Drug Administration safety alert based on 38 reports of "life-threatening" complications when Infuse was used in neck surgeries, an unapproved use, received over 4 years (FDA 2008). Since then, Infuse has been linked to sterility in men, cancer (Wilson and Meier 2009) and other serious complications (Fauber 2012a, b, c). In 2012, a 16-month congressional investigation found that Medtronic "paid a total of approximately $210 million to physician authors of Medtronic-sponsored studies" in 14 years and "violate[d] the trust patients have in their medical care."

Interventional Pain Management

Early efforts at interventional pain date all the way back to 1899 when the first therapeutic nerve block was described in France (Manchikanti et al. 2003). Today, interventional pain medicine is a thriving subspecialty of pain management that encompasses techniques that include epidural injections, epidural and root blocks, facet injections and medical branch blocks, sympathetic blocks, spinal cord stimulation, and radio-frequency denervation (also called nerve ablation or "burning").

Interventional pain techniques are analogous to surgery in that their outcome is partially dependent on the experience and skill of the operator. While growing in popularity, especially in the United States, there is "insufficient data to speak for the efficacy of many…commonly performed procedures" (Zhao and Cope 2013). Other limitations to interventional pain techniques are the pain relief is short-lived, there is the risk of complications, sometimes serious and "pain reduction does not necessarily translate into improved function and return to work." Nonetheless, American spent $23 billion on interventional pain techniques in 2011, including epidurals, implants of spinal cord stimulators, and injections of painkillers (Armstrong 2011). Interventional pain techniques have grown by 231 % since 2002.

Injections/Nerve Blocks

The use of injections for chronic pain, whether corticosteroids, anesthetic painkillers or both, increased by 159 % between 2000 and 2010 in Medicare patients with 9 million Americans receiving pain injections in 2010 alone (Armstrong 2011). The surge was driven by the aging of the US population and the financial remuneration behind the injections themselves. Epidural injections, which deliver corticosteroid via a catheter into the space between the dura and the spine, are especially popular. Medicare paid about $200 for a typical epidural steroid injection given in a physician's office, $400 for the procedure at a surgery center and about $600 when performed at a hospital.

Despite their wide use, the efficacy of epidural is not overwhelming as we see in Table 5.3. "Data addressing the effects of epidural steroid injection on pain from spinal stenosis, low back pain without radicular pain and failed back surgery is sparse" and "no long-term efficacy of epidural procedures for chronic spinal pain has been established," say Zhao and Cope in Springer's *Handbook of Pain and Palliative Care* (2013). Guidelines from the American Society of Anesthesiologists, American Pain Society, the American Academy of Pain, the American College of Occupational and Environmental Medicine and the American Society of Interventional Pain Physicians concur that epidural injections with or without local anesthetics provide pain relief from 2 weeks to 3 months but that the magnitude of their pain reduction is "modest."

In 2014, the *New England Journal of Medicine* published an article and editorial questioning the benefit of using steroid injections for spinal stenosis at all (Friedly et al. 2014). Six weeks of injections with a steroid and the anesthetic lidocaine were no more effective than injections with lidocaine, said researchers. "This study shows that the steroid is not the reason why patients are getting this significant relief. It could just be the lidocaine itself," Dr. Nick Shamie of the UCLA Spine

Table 5.3 Limitations of epidural injections

Short-term pain relief (a few weeks)
Little improvement of function
Do not obviate need for surgery
Stroke, paralysis among risks
Quality problems from pharmacies

Center explained (CBS 2014). The journal's conclusion angered interventional pain physicians who wrote that there were "severe limitations to this study, manuscript, and accompanying editorial. The design, inclusion criteria, outcomes assessment, analysis of data and interpretation, and conclusions of this trial point to the fact that this highly sophisticated and much publicized randomized trial may not be appropriate and lead to misinformation" (Manchikanti et al. 2014a, b).

But others echoed the efficacy doubts. "In general, epidural steroid injection for radicular lumbosacral pain does not impact average impairment of function, need for surgery, or provide long-term pain relief beyond 3 months," concluded a report of the Therapeutics and Technology Assessment Subcommittee of the American Academy of Neurology in the journal *Neurology* (Armon et al. 2007). "Their routine use for these indications is not recommended."

Two of the nation's leading pain specialists, Roger Chou, M.D. and John D. Loeser, M.D., write in an American Pain Society guideline that steroid injections for discogenic back pain and intra-articular facet joint pain are "not effective, nor is prolotherapy," injecting a nonactive irritant into the body to try to lessen pain (Chou et al. 2009).

Unlike some studies which suggest patients experienced a drop in pain for several weeks after an epidural steroid injection, in one study, epidural steroids didn't surpass placebo in relieving back pain at 24 h, 3 or 6 months. Nor did the epidurals improve back function or allow patients to avoid subsequent back surgery (Hitti 2007). "While some pain relief is a positive result in and of itself, the extent of leg and back pain relief from epidural steroid injections, on the average, fell short of the values typically viewed as clinically meaningful," said Carmel Armon, M.D. of Tufts University's medical school about the study (American Academy of Neurology 2007).

In 2012 and 2013, steroid injections came under major scrutiny when at least 63 people died from fungal meningitis caused by contamination of the injection liquid (Lubell 2013). The preservative-free injections, made by loosely regulated compounding pharmacies, sickened people in 10 states including 264 people in Michigan alone (Zaniewski 2013). The FDA subsequently tightened regulations on compounding pharmacies, refining manufacturing standards and the list of drugs considered too risky to be altered. Sanctions against compounding pharmacies which did not comply were also strengthened (Al-Faruque 2014).

But even before the fungal meningitis outbreak, 78 cases of patients sustaining injuries from steroid injections were recorded in the journal *Spine* in 2007 (Armstrong 2013) including 13 deaths and cases of loss of vision, stroke, and paralysis. Richard Rosenquist, M.D. chairman of the pain management department at the prestigious Cleveland Clinic, called the complications, "devastating" (Armstrong 2011).

In 2014, the FDA cautioned that injection of corticosteroids into the epidural space of the spine may cause "loss of vision, stroke, paralysis, and death," a warning that interventional pain physicians also disputed, citing inaccuracies (Manchikanti et al. 2014a, b). Epidural injections, with or without steroids, are effective "in a multitude of spinal ailments utilizing caudal, cervical, thoracic, and lumbar interlaminar approaches as well as lumbar transforaminal epidural injections," maintained practitioners. "The evidence also shows the superiority of steroids in managing lumbar disk herniation utilizing caudal and lumbar interlaminar approaches without any significant difference as compared to transforaminal approaches, either with local anesthetic alone or local anesthetic and steroids combined." Three authors cited financial links to medical device makers including Medtronic.

Spinal Cord Stimulators

As back surgery has increased, especially in the United States, so has the number of patients suffering from failed back surgery or FBSS. In attempts to treat FBSS non-surgically, spinal cord stimulation (SCS), a technique first developed over 50 years ago, has been growing in popularity. The process involves the careful placement of electrode leads into the epidural space, followed by a trial period to predict outcome. If the trial period proves to be effective, the leads are anchored, a pulse generator or radio-frequency receiver is implanted and connection wires are tunneled and connected.

Spinal cord stimulation was originally based on Melzack and Wall's 1965 Gate Theory that proposed that stimulation of innocuous neural pathways, carried on large C-fibers could block concurrent noxious information carried on faster moving A-delta fibers, effectively "closing the gate" on CNS pain (Lee and Vasudevan 2012). However, the actual neurophysiologic mechanism of action may be more complex than originally postulated. For example, pain reduction may result from direct inhibition of pain transmission in the dorsal horn of the spinal cord and possible recruitment of endogenous inhibitory pathways through the posterior columns of the spinal cord. One reason to believe other mechanisms may be at play in SCS besides those detailed in the Gate Theory is that pain relief may last several hours after cessation of the actual spine stimulation. This suggests long-lasting modulation of neural activity at the level of local transmitter systems in the dorsal horn.

In fact, the neurophysiologic mechanism of SCS suggests a simultaneous increase in GABA and serotonin with concurrent suppression of glutamate and aspartate. Research with antidepressants such as milnacipran or amitriptyline suggests the N-methyl-D-aspartate receptor, which effects the induction and maintenance of neuropathic pain, may be involved in SCS pain reduction. In Chap. 6, Treating the Chronic Pain Patient, we explore the use of drugs such as antidepressants and anti-seizure medications in seeking to treat nerves involved in modulating chronic pain.

Significantly, SCS does not treat nociceptive pain effectively, lending more credence to theories that neurotransmitter activity is also involved in SCS actions. Studies have shown that SCS is able to dampen both continuous and evoked pain (tactile/thermal allodynia), but has had little effect on induced, acute nociceptive pain. This is a limitation of SCS, as an only 10–19 % of chronic pain is estimated to be characterized with neuropathic pain (Lee and Vasudevan 2012).

While evidence supports SCS's ability to reduce pain by at least 50 %, it does not guarantee pain relief in all patients and outcome depends on careful patient selection.

Table 5.4 Factors
affecting SCS outcomes
in patients

The significance patient attributes to a pain condition
Expectation of pain; amplified pain sensitivity
Feelings of lack of control and uncertainty, social isolation
The view that the patient's culture has on painful experiences
Coexisting anxiety and depression
Other coexisting psychopathologies

For example the following factors presented by a patient predict a poor outcome when using spinal cord stimulation as shown in Table 5.4.

Like any invasive procedure, SCS carries the risk of complications. Thirty-four percent of patients who received a spinal cord stimulator experienced complications in one study, with the most common complications being electrode migration (11 %), lead fracture (6 %), infection (5 %), hardware malfunction (2.5 %), and discomfort over the generator implant site and rotation of the generator (2.5 %).

Twenty-six to 32 % of patients receiving spine stimulators "experienced a complication following spinal cord stimulator implantation, including electrode migration, infection or wound breakdown, generator pocket-related complications, and lead problems" (Lee and Vasudevan 2012) said an article in *Pain Management*. Medtronic lists risks with its implantable neurostimulation system as hematoma, epidural hemorrhage, paralysis, seroma, CSF leakage, infection, erosion, allergic response, hardware malfunction or migration, pain at implant site, loss of pain relief, and chest wall stimulation.

Finally, spinal cord stimulation is a labor-intensive and expensive procedure with out-of-pocket costs ranging from $15,000 to over $50,000 and considerable additional expenses for annual maintenance. It is clearly not for a wide swath of patients and results have been mixed among my own patients over the years.

Radio-Frequency Denervation

Perhaps no treatment so well demonstrates the puzzle of chronic pain and the difficulty so many theories have in fully explaining it as radio-frequency denervation, also called ablation or "nerve burning." Despite destruction of the nerves that are apparently involved in a patient's pain, the pain sensations often persist—and can migrate to new loci and/or intensify. The existence of this paradox, which seems an anatomical impossibility, brings to mind phantom pain which Melzack and Wall note even exists in people born without the limbs in which they "feel" pain. Clearly the brain is involved in such mediations since there could be no "memory" of the limb existing or its neural pathways.

Radio-frequency denervation or ablation, most commonly used for neck or back pain caused by arthritis or injury, interrupts nerves going directly to individual facet joints thus blocking the sympathetic nerve supply. It is also used for arms or legs affected by complex regional pain syndrome (CRPS) and for degenerative disks, occipital neuralgia, and certain types of abdominal pain. CRPS and other specific pain disorders are addressed in Chap. 10.

Most patients who consider radio-frequency denervation have tried anti-inflammatory medication and physical therapy with limited success and have responded well to diagnostic or trial injections to predict effectiveness of denervation.

Denervation can be accomplished through surgical destruction of the nerves like rhizotomy, cordotomy, and tractotomy, "burning" nerves with radio frequency or electrical current or treating the nerves with the drug phenol. Like other interventional treatments in which the target nerves cannot actually be seen (transforaminal, interlaminar and caudal epidurals, medial branch blocks) X-ray or fluoroscopy is used to guide placement of the introducer needles and identify bony landmarks.

Nerve conduction can be blocked using denervation on a permanent basis or semi-permanent basis (as short as 3 months) or as long as 18 months or longer. But, after brief periods of relief, pain often recurs in patients and new and abnormal pain sensations sometimes also occur. *Drs. Chou and Loeser write that there is "poor evidence" of the effectiveness of radio-frequency denervation on presumed discogenic, facet joint or radiculopathic pain* (Chou et al. 2009).

Complications are also possible since the nerves to be ablated may be near blood vessels or other nerves that can be damaged and electrical current used during the procedure can cause an electrical burn. Denervation, when used for facet joint pain, can also produce allergic reactions, infection, rupture of a tendon and depigmentation and thinning of the affected skin (Zylberger 2009).

Non-evidence-Based Care Often Not Cost-Effective

As new pain intervention techniques have surfaced in developed countries in the last decades, especially the United States, and become highly profitable, "pill mills" and "pain clinics" have also proliferated. While some attempt to acknowledge the many facets to pain and a patient's complex pain treatment history (treating the "person" and not the "pain"), many are unabashedly profit centers seeking volume and return "business."

Pill mills dispensing opioid painkillers with few questions asked usually require no appointments, handle no insurance and give only cursory attention to medical records and physical examinations. Some even have armed guards which is the ultimate "tip off." Interventional pain clinics can also be mills with "shot jocks" routinely dispensing injections/nerve blocks with little attention to a patient's long-term outcomes. In Chap. 8, Creating a Multidisciplinary Team, we discuss the features that distinguish legitimate pain centers from profiteering pill or "shot" mills. We also discuss how you can develop your own virtual rehabilitation team when bricks and mortar facilities are lacking.

As the Affordable Care Act (ACA), also called Obamacare, regulated some payments for interventional pain care, especially Medicare reimbursements, the interventional pain medicine industry vigorously fought back. The American Society of Interventional Pain Physicians estimated that 40 % of its practitioners would cease their practice because of drops in reimbursements under ACA. The medical group also threatened that "suffering" and hospitalizations would increase and opioid painkillers "may be the only option" for their chronic pain patients, if reimbursements are cut for interventional techniques (Silverman 2014).

Yet refusing outsized Medicare reimbursements for pain interventions that are not evidence-based may not be such a bad thing. Contrary to industry pushback, the alternative to injections and nerve blocks does not need to be opioid painkillers except when patients are unadvisedly seeking an instant "cure" or "quick fix" to their pain—and medical professionals willing to oblige them.

Multidisciplinary pain rehabilitation programs, which were the effective and cost-effective treatment for chronic pain before the surgery and interventional medicine emphasis, hopefully will come back into vogue. Certainly, they require an initial investment for the time and expertise of allied professionals like physical and occupational therapists and health psychologists; certainly they call for more work and patience on the part of both patients and clinicians than unimodal and "quick fix" treatment. But the long-term outcomes of multidisciplinary pain programs, especially outside of the United States where they flourish, outperform less evidence-based, unimodal techniques whether excessive surgeries, interventions or long-term prescription of opioids. All these popular treatments address the biologically-caused symptoms of pain while disregarding the psychological factors behind chronic pain that are continually described in the literature. For that reason, they are often minimally effective in relieving patients' pain and often have to be repeated.

Opioid Drugs

Opioid painkillers have been invaluable in treating acute pain after injury and surgery for hundreds of years. (Opiates and synthetic opioids are frequently referred to as "narcotics" which is actually a legal not medical term.) Opioids allow medical professionals to provide comfort to terminally ill patients and patients suffering from cancer and other painful conditions. They are a vital and irreplaceable important component of "palliative care." *But physicians are increasingly divided about the use of opioid in the treatment of chronic pain.*

In a sense, the "pendulum" about the advisability and safety of opioids for chronic pain has swung back not once but twice. Before the 1960s and 1970s when pain was regarded as a purely physiological occurrence and before multidisciplinary developed, opioids were often prescribed for relief of pain despite their addictive potential. As problems with addiction and diversion surfaced, regulations were put in place to restrict the use of opioids and tighten their control. In the 1990s, the pendulum again swung back, thanks to popular new opioids like OxyContin, online drug sales and high-level marketing by drug companies. In the 1990s, opioids began to be prescribed "for a new use: treating long-term pain from back injuries, headaches, arthritis and conditions like fibromyalgia" (Meier 2013).

One example was the American Geriatrics Society which changed its guidelines in 2009 to recommend "that over-the-counter pain relievers, such as ibuprofen and naproxen, be used rarely and that doctors instead consider prescribing opioids for all patients with moderate to severe pain" (Fauber and Gabler 2012a, b). Half the panel's experts "had financial ties to opioid companies, as paid speakers, consultants or advisers at the time the guidelines were issued," Fauber reports. The University of Wisconsin's Pain & Policy Studies Group also took $2.5 million from opioid makers even as it pushed for looser use of narcotic painkillers, he reports.

A pain guide called *Finding Relief: Pain Management for Older Adults*, endorsed by the American Geriatrics Society and funded by the drug company PriCara (which mas the opioid products Duragesic, Ultram ER and Nucynta and became Janssen) claims that opioids "allow people with chronic pain to get back to work, run, and play sports," according to Medpage and describes as worries that patients may need increased doses of opioids over time as a "myth". While omitting established opioid risks, the guide did cite "disadvantages" for ibuprofen (Advil) and naproxen (Aleve).

Another example was the lobbying of FDA decision makers by a drug company-funded group called IMMPACT whose stated goal is "improving the design, execution, and interpretation of clinical trials of treatments for pain." One of the improved designs it recommends is "enriched enrollment"—elimination of nonresponders and subjects who don't tolerate a drug before the clinical trial begins. Both Purdue Pharma, which makes OxyContin, and Janssen, which makes the opioids Duragesic and Nucynta, have acknowledged the value of IMMPACT's efforts to improve clinical trial procedures which of course lowers drug company trial costs while heightening the chance a drug candidate is approved (Rosenberg 2014).

Many physicians and medical groups also downplayed the drugs' dangers, either because they received heavily marketed promotions or because they had not seen patients with opioid-related problems for a long time. In either case, there was a collective and incorrect impression in much of the medical community that opioid drugs were not dangerous anymore.

Yet opioids are far from benign. They cause hormonal changes (decreases in testosterone), constipation, a decrease in immune responses and, of course, tolerance progressing toward physical dependence and addiction. In *Responsible Opioid Prescribing*, Dr. Scott Fishman also lists "heightened fracture risk related to effects and bone metabolism and from falls," and increased risks for the elderly and "those with impaired renal or hepatic function; individuals with cardiopulmonary disorders, such as chronic obstructive pulmonary disease (COPD); congestive heart failure (CHF), sleep apnea, or mental illness; and in patients who combine opioids with other respiratory depressants such as alcohol, sedative-hypnotics, benzodiazepines, or barbiturates" (2012).

Paradoxically, opioids used for more than a short period of time can *increase* sensitivity to pain—a well recognized syndrome called Opioid Induced Hypersensitivity

(OIH). Many patients report, to their surprise, their pain subsides when they cease their long-term use of opioids. There is little evidence that opioids are effective after 6 weeks and a concerning dearth of long-term studies (Fauber 2015).

Opioid limitations
Addictive potential
Overdose/drug interactions/deaths
Limited or no long-term pain relief
Limited or no functional improvement seen
Increase in pain (Opioid-Induced Hypersensitivity)
Psychological changes in mood; risk of depression
Falls and accidents from impaired balance and cognition
Fractures from Impaired Bone Metabolism
Psychological changes—passivity helplessness
Hormonal/Endocrine impairment
Immune impairment
Constipation
Risks in renal and hepatic patients
Risks in COPD and CHF patients
Risks with mental patients
Impaired judgment

Nor are opioids always associated with improvement in function. As we saw in Chap. 2, workers who received high opioid doses actually stayed out of work three times longer in a California study and experienced "delayed recovery from workplace injuries" (Meier 2013).

Workers kept on opioids for more than 7 days during the first 6 weeks after an injury were more than twice as likely to be disabled and out of work a year later, according to a *Spine* study (Fauber and Gabler 2012a, b) and in a large study always Workers' Compensation claims neither pain nor function improved with opioid use. In an earlier study in *Spine*, workers who received early opioid drugs in morphine equivalent amounts of more than 450 mg "were, on average, disabled 69 days longer than those who received no early opioids" and their "risk for surgery was three times greater" (Webster et al. 2007). "Given the negative association between receipt of early opioids for acute LBP and outcomes, it is suggested that the use of opioids for the management of acute LBP may be counterproductive to recovery," the study concludes.

In 2013, Johnson & Johnson, the parent company of Janssen who makes the opioid patch Duragesic and Nucynta, an oral opioid was investigated by the city of Chicago for deceptively marketing the drugs to city employees for long-term treatment of chronic pain, such as back pain and arthritis (Morris 2013).

Elderly patients have especially been harmed by overprescription of opioid drugs (Eisler 2014). "Older brains and bodies are prone to drug complications, from falls and respiratory failure to cognitive problems and dementia," and "because older bodies metabolize drugs less quickly, those medications tend to build up in their bodies" said an expose in *USA Today* in 2014. Still, "one in every four adults 50 and over use psychoactive medications—mostly opioids for pain" despite the fact that 75 % of pharmaceutical overdose deaths involved opioid painkillers, according to CDC data (*USA Today*).

Opioid Crisis Underway

We are now in the midst of a chilling opioid abuse epidemic which is playing out both in prescription drugs like oxycodone, hydrocodone, fentanyl, hydromorphone, morphine and methadone, and in the use of street drugs like heroin. The latter is attributed to people who became addicted to pills which they could no longer afford or procure, driving them to street drugs.

More than 17,000 people die in the United States every year from opioid overdoses and emergency room admissions for opioids (other than heroin) went from 299,000 in 2001 to 885,000 in 2011 (Aleccia 2013). Poisonings from opioids, legal drugs (alcohol) and illegal drugs (heroin, cocaine), now lead car accidents in injury deaths and 90 % are from drugs, mostly painkillers (Fauber 2012a, b, c).

Thanks to the second swing of the pendulum, opioid painkillers soon were prescribed for almost every pain condition. They "didn't discriminate among the causes of human suffering—be it back pain, fibromyalgia, toothaches, cancer, depression, divorce, boredom, mental illness, unemployment, hip replacement, or withdrawal symptoms" (Gilette 2012). Sadly, one Florida mill lured 12 physicians to work in its operation. Physicians could earn $37,500 a week—at $100 per prescription.

Florida was far from the only place that medical professionals participated in the opioid racket. In 2014, former director of pharmacy services for Beth Israel Medical Center in New York City, was arrested and charged with stealing and illegally possessing oxycodone with a street value of almost $5.6 million (Pain Medicine News 2014).

Santa Clara County, in California, sued the drug companies Purdue Pharma, Cephalon, Janssen Pharmaceuticals, Endo Health Solutions and Actavis for allegedly addicting Californians to prescription opioids for profit in 2014 (Mintz 2014). "Defendants' deceptive marketing campaign deprived California patients and their doctors of the ability to make informed medical decisions and, instead, caused important, sometimes life-or-death decisions to be made based not on science, but hype," the lawsuit alleged. Assistant Santa Clara County Counsel Danny Chou accused the drug companies of a "decades-long marketing plan…to create a market for these drugs that never should have existed" which "spawned a new generation of addicts and abusers" (Rucke 2014). Chou also charged opioid makers with secretly funding advocacy organizations like the American Pain Foundation which, he said, appear to be independent but are actually promoting opioids.

Abuse of opioids has also worked its way into the sports world. In 2014, the Drug Enforcement Administration (DEA) launched an investigation into opioid misuse within the National Football League after attorneys representing about 1300 NFL retirees filed a class-action lawsuit (O'Keefe 2014). The NFL illegally provided prescription painkillers to keep players on the field without informing them of the long-term risks, charged the suit.

Growing alongside the pill mills has been another industry—"opioid addiction" treatment clinics which dispense narcotic agonists like Suboxone, a combination of buprenorphine and naloxone. "Subs" and "Bupe" are booming in popularity on the street to treat addiction to opioids called "Oxies" and "Roxies" and for the "highs" they also create. There is currently a growth industry in the business of selling Suboxone which raises concern that so-called addiction treatment clinics are now part of the problem.

One reason for the booming opioid abuse epidemic was the introduction of long-acting opioids like OxyContin. Initially, the pills solved three problems that had been associated with short-acting opioid drugs. Because short-acting drugs, which are taken as needed, require 20–30 min to work and last only 2–4 h, the patient's peak of pain is often missed. This can lead patients to exceed their doses and risk abuse and toxicity. Secondly, most short-acting opioids are combined with acetaminophen (Tylenol) which causes liver damage at high doses. Long-acting opioids lacked Tylenol so if patients had to take "rescue doses" of short-acting opioids for "breakthrough" pain, there were less risks. Finally, short-acting opioids taken as needed encourage "reward-seeking," addictive behavior and make patients focus on their pain. For all these reasons, long-acting opioids, taken on a time-contingent basis like one at 7 a.m. and one at 7 p.m., were believed to be an improvement on pain control.

But of course recreational drug users and drug abusers soon found they could crush and snort long-acting opioids and even shoot them like heroin. This allowed people to take all 80 mg in an OxyContin pill at one time which was a "rush" they described as better than cocaine. Once the "snort and shoot" potential was discovered, the street value of opioids went from $4 to $5 dollars per pill to $1 a milligram or $40 to $80 per pill.

As the full impact of the opioid addiction epidemic became apparent, taking as many as 60 lives a day in the United States, both drug companies and drug regulators began to act. In 2013, the Food and Drug Administration (FDA) responded to the epidemic by removing the "moderate pain" indication found on their labels and restricting the drugs to severe pain (Lowes 2013). In addition, based on concerns that Vicodin, with the active ingredient hydrocodone, has been the most prescribed drug in the United States (99 % of the world's hydrocodone is used by the 4.5 % of the world, people in the United States), the FDA considered moving the medication from a Schedule III drug to a Schedule II drug. Schedule III drugs do not require a physician visit to obtain a prescription whereas Schedule II drugs do. The latter, like oxycodone and morphine, are also limited to a 30-day supply.

Manufacturers complied with new FDA directives and created abuse-proof versions of long-acting opioids, like OxyContin which had driven so much abuse. In 2014, the FDA-approved Targiniq ER, an opioid pain reliever said to be the first to combine oxycodone with naloxone hydrochloride to block the euphoric effects that drive addiction and abuse. But even the FDA admitted that euphoric effects of oxy-codone are blocked if the drug is crushed and snorted or injected but not if the drug is taken orally and that overdoses can still occur (FDA 2014). Moreover, other opioids, like fentanyl, Actiq, and the more recent long-acting hydrocodone (Zydone) are *not* abuse-deterrent and public health officials and pain experts are baffled by the FDA's apparent tin ear to the national opioid problem.

Several of the leaders in the field of pain medicine/pain management who believed that high doses of opioids could be an answer for treating chronic pain have, over the years, expressed regret later in promoting this approach to treatment. Russell Portenoy, M.D. from the Mount Sinai Health System in New York is a leader in the pain field but, after almost three decades of promoting the use of opioids, reversed his position and spoke out about their negative impact on patients, families, and society (Catan and Pereza 2012). The American Academy of Pain Medicine (AAPM) has pledged to "reduce deaths and other adverse events related to the use of prescription opioids in the treatment of chronic pain, while preserving access for appropriately selected pain patients" (2014).

The highly respected Cochrane Collection wrote in 2014 that "There are no placebo-RCTs supporting the effectiveness and safety of long-term opioid therapy for treatment of CLBP (chronic low back pain)" and that "The initiation of a trial of opioids for long-term management should be done with extreme caution, especially after a comprehensive assessment of potential risks." Cochrane also noted that, "The very few trials that compared opioids to non-steroidal anti-inflammatory drugs (NSAIDs) or antidepressants did not show any differences regarding pain and function."

The Federation of State Medical Boards (FSMB) has also reviewed the use of opioids and issued a new policy in 2013 about when and how to use them in patients with chronic pain. No longer is there a blank check to prescribe the drugs. Instead, according to the new policy, there must be a diagnosis of what is believed to be causing the pain, a delineation of specific functional goals that can be accomplished with opioid use and acceptance of responsibility on the part of physicians and prescribers to prevent diversion and abuse. A book by Scott Fishman, M.D. a past president of the American Academy of Pain Medicine (AAPM) and the American Pain Foundation who has also authored a related book, *Responsible Opioid Prescribing-A Clinician's Guide*, republished in 2012 is also recommended by FSMB and other state Medical Examining Boards.

The government has also cracked down on the vast opioid networks using online pharmacies. Shipping giants Federal Express and United Parcel Service were both sued in 2014 by federal prosecutors for knowingly delivering "controlled substances and prescription drugs from online pharmacies to individuals who subsequently died or accidentally caused the death of others" (Elias 2014).

The opioid epidemic blurred the lines between "real" pain patients, false "patients" reselling drugs and "real" patients who became addicted through the medical care they were given. Pain clinics and pill operations "cut off" such patients despite often being largely responsible for their habituation. This is a classic example of blaming the victim. "The problem is patients are started, develop tolerance, need a higher dose, get tolerant to the higher dose, use more than prescribed, ask for early refills, get switched to a 'pain management specialist,' who if they violate the pain contracts, get fired, discharged, and then they go to the street for the opioids," says James O'Donnell, a pharmacology professor at Rush University in Chicago.

Table 5.5 Main points of this chapter

Uncoordinated, unimodal treatments for chronic pain predominate
Spine surgeries, especially fusions are overused and have mixed outcomes
Interventions/epidurals offer only short-term benefits
Spinal cord stimulators and nerve ablation present limitations
Long-term opioids not effective—overdoses and diversions are seen
Unimodal treatments less cost-effective than multidisciplinary care because of failure rates

In Chap. 6, Treating the Chronic Pain Patient, effective, multidisciplinary treatments that blend many modalities will be discussed. In Chap. 8, you will learn how to assemble a multidisciplinary team or virtual team of allied health professionals, near where you practice.

References

Abaci, P. (2010). *Take charge of your chronic pain*. New York: GPP Life.

Abelson, R., & Petersen, M. (2003, December 31). An operation to ease back pain bolsters the bottom line, too. *New York Times*.

Aleccia, J. (2013, July 2). Opiate overdose deaths 'skyrocketed' in women, CDC finds. *NBC News*.

Al-Faruque, F. (2014, July 1). FDA tightens oversight of pharmacies. *The Hill*.

American Academy of Neurology. (2007, March 5). *New guideline: Epidural steroid injections limited in treating back pain*. Press release.

American Pain Society. (2007). *Guidelines for the evaluation and management of low back pain evidence review*. Glenview, IL: American Pain Society.

Armon, C., Argoff, C., Samuels, J., et al. (2007). Report of the therapeutics and technology assessment subcommittee of the assessment: Use of epidural steroid injections to treat radicular lumbosacral pain. *Neurology, 68*, 723–729.

Armstrong, D. (2011, December 27). Epidurals linked to paralysis seen with $300 billion pain market. *Bloomberg*.

Armstrong, D. (2013, April 25). FDA warning on pain injections comes too late for some. *Bloomberg Businessweek*.

Blaszczak-Boxe, G. (2014, June 30). Are doctors performing too many unnecessary knee-replacement surgeries? *CBS News*.

Brawley, O. (2011). *How we do harm*. New York: St. Martins.

Brownlee, S. (2007, October). Newtered. *Washington Monthly*.

Catan, T., & Pereza, E. (2012, December 15). Pain-drug champion has second thoughts. *Wall Street Journal*.

CBS News (2014, July 2). Dr. Max Gomez: New study questions the effectiveness of epidural injections.

Chou, R., Loeser, J., Owens, D., Rosenquist, R., Atlas, S., Baisden, J., et al. (2009). Interventional therapies, surgery, and interdisciplinary rehabilitation for low back pain. *Spine, 34*(10), 1066–1077.

Deyo, R., & Mirza, S. (2009). The case for restraint in spinal surgery. *European Spine Journal, 18*(Suppl. 3), 331–337.

Eisler, P. (2014, May 22). Older Americans hooked on Rx. *USA Today*.

Elias, P. (2014, August 15). Money laundering charge added to FedEx drug case. *Associated Press*.

Fauber, J. (2011, December 26). Medtronic paid millions to influential UW chairman. *Journal-Sentinel*.

Fauber, J. (2012a, May 29). Narcotics use for chronic pain soars among seniors. *Journal Sentinel*.

Fauber, J. (2012b, October 2). Many injured workers remain on opioids, study finds. *Milwaukee Journal Sentinel*.

Fauber, J. (2012c, October 25). Medtronic helped write, edit positive 'Infuse' spine studies. *Medpage Today*.

Fauber, J. (2015, January 12). Studies find little evidence of benefit from long-term opioid use. Most clinical trials haven't gone beyond 6 weeks. *Milwaukee Journal Sentinel*.

Fauber, J., & Gabler, E. (2012a, May 29). Experts linked to drug firms tout benefits but downplay chance of addiction, other risks. *Milwaukee Journal Sentinel*.

Fauber, J., & Gabler, E. (2012b, May 30). Narcotic painkiller use booming among elderly. *Milwaukee Journal Sentinel/Medpage*.

FDA. (2008, July 1). Life-threatening complications associated with recombinant human bone morphogenetic protein in cervical spine fusion. Public Health Notification.

FDA. (2014, July 23). FDA approves new extended-release oxycodone with abuse-deterrent properties. Press release.

Fishman, S. (2012). *Responsible opioid prescribing*. Washington, DC: Waterford Life Sciences.

Food and Drug Administration. (2014, April 23). Drug Safety Communication: FDA requires label changes to warn of rare but serious neurologic problems after epidural corticosteroid injections for pain.

Friedly, J., et al. (2014). A randomized trial of epidural glucocorticoid injections for spinal stenosis. *New England Journal of Medicine, 371*, 11–21.

Gilette, F. (2012, June 6). American pain: The largest U.S. pill mill's rise and fall. *Businessweek*.

Groopman, J. (2007). *How doctors think*. New York: Houghton Mifflin.

Hadler, N. (2008). *Worried sick* (pp. 118–123). Chapel Hill: University of North Carolina Press.

Hitti, M. (2007, March 5). Steroid shots for back pain don't work. Professional group advises against epidural steroid shots for chronic back pain. *WebMD*.

Institute of Medicine. (2011). *Relieving pain in America*. Washington, DC: The National Academies Press.

International Association for the Study of Pain. (2013, June). *Insight*, pp. 19–20. Academies Press.

Lee, N., & Vasudevan, S. (2012). Spinal cord stimulation use in patients with failed back surgery syndrome. *Pain Manage, 2*(2), 135–140.

Lowes, R. (2013, September 10). FDA restricts long-term opioid use to combat abuse. *Medscape*.

Lubell, J. (2013, August 12). Groundwork laid for lawsuits over deaths from tainted steroids. *American Medical News*.

Manchikanti, L., Boswell, M., Raj, P., & Racz, G. (2003). The evolution of interventional pain management. *Pain Physician, 6*, 485–494.

Manchikanti, L., Candido, K., Kaye, A., Boswell, M., Benyamin, R., Falco, F., Gharibo, C., & Hirsch, J. (2014a). Randomized trial of epidural injections for spinal stenosis published in the New England Journal of Medicine: Further confusion without clarification. *Pain Physician, 17*, E475–E487.

Manchikanti, L., Candido, K., Singh, V., Gharibo, C., Boswell, M., Benyamin, R., et al. (2014b). Epidural steroid warning controversy still dogging FDA. *Pain Physician, 17*(4), E451–E474.

Medtronic. (2014). *Indications, safety, and warnings. Medtronic implantable neurostimulation system*. Retrieved from http://professional.medtronic.com/pt/neuro/scs/ind/index.htm#.Up9zl2AYhe4

Meier, B. (2013, June 23). Profiting from pain. *New York Times*.

Melzack, R., & Wall, P. (1988). *The challenge of pain*. New York: Penguin Books.

Mintz, H. (2014, May 22). Santa Clara County sues drug makers for hyping painkillers. *San Jose Mercury News*.

Morris, M. (2013, November 14). Emanuel administration probes J&J unit over drug marketing. *Crains*.

O'Keefe, M. (2014, July 12). Feds quietly investigating prescription drug abuse in NFL locker. *New York Daily News*.

Pain Medicine News. (2014, April). Case of large-scale opioid diversion puts hospitals on alert.

Pear, R. (2014, August 16). Medicare to start paying doctors who coordinate needs of chronically ill patients. *New York Times*.

Rosenberg, M. (2014, May 15). How big pharma and the FDA drive the opioid addiction epidemic. *Reporting on Health*. University of Southern California.

Rucke, K. (2014, July 9). California, Chicago sue addictive painkiller manufacturers. *MintPress News*. Retrieved from http://www.mintpressnews.com/california-chicago-sue-addictive-painkiller-manufacturers/193660/

Silverman. S. (2014, January 5). Costs to manage pain will go up under Obamacare. *Sun Sentinel*.

The American Academy of Pain Medicine. (2014). *AAPM's 2013 safe opioid prescribing initiative*. Retrieved from http://www.painmed.org/safeprescribing/

U.S. Senate (2012, October 25). *Baucus-Grassley investigation into medtronic reveals manipulated studies, close financial ties with researchers, committee on finance*. Retrieved from http://www.finance.senate.gov/newsroom/chairman/release/?id=b1d112cb-230f-4c2e-ae55-13550074fe86

Webster, B., Verma, S. K., & Gatchel, R. J. (2007). Relationship between early opioid prescribing for acute occupational low back pain and disability duration, medical costs, subsequent surgery and late opioid use. *Spine, 32*(19), 2127–2132.

Wells-Federman, C. L. (1999). Care of the patient with chronic pain: Part I. *Clinical Excellence for Nurse Practitioners, 3*(4), 192–204.

Wheeler, A. et al. (2013, January 8). Low back pain and sciatica. *Medscape*.

Wilson, D., & Meier, B. (2009, May 12). Doctor falsified study on injured G.I.'s, Army says. *New York Times*.

Zaniewski, A. (2013, July 29). Two more Michigan deaths linked to tainted steroid injections. *Detroit Free Press*.

Zhao, Z., & Cope, D. K. (2013). Nerve blocks, trigger points, and intrathecal therapy for chronic pain. In R. Moore (Ed.), *Handbook of pain and palliative care* (pp. 550–556). Rockville, MD: Springer.

Zylberger, D. (2009). *Facet pain and radiofrequency ablation*. Presentation. New York-Presbyterian. Retrieved from http://nyp.org/pdf/1050_Zylberger.pdf

Chapter 6
Treating the Chronic Pain Patient

How I Came to Embrace Multidisciplinary Treatment

Since the age of four, I wanted to be a physician and I had expected to become an orthopedic surgeon, as I was always interested in the function of bones, joints, and muscles. Later, my interest was also in the nervous system and its control of the musculoskeletal system. I emigrated to the United States in 1973, after finishing my medical school training in India, and undertook a year of surgical training in Honolulu, Hawaii. However, I did not find surgery as rewarding as I had anticipated. By serendipity, I met a physiatrist in 1973 who suggested I consider the field of physical medicine and rehabilitation, a specialty that would let me care for individuals with a variety of musculoskeletal and neurological disabilities.

I soon began a residency in Physical Medicine & Rehabilitation at the medical college of Wisconsin in Milwaukee. This work and the knowledge I gained as I pursued certifications by various pain medicine related boards, strengthened my belief in the value of a multidisciplinary approach to pain management. Chronic pain, a condition in which pain lasts beyond the normal healing period, has no clear cause or cure and is associated with disability and often depression and drug misuse, is ideally suited for a multidisciplinary approach because it addresses the multiple psychosocial and biologic factors behind it. As we noted in the introduction to this book, multidisciplinary rehabilitation with its team of medical professionals who are experts in their varying fields treats the "person" not the pain.

During this same time period, I was becoming trained in the disability systems in the United States and performing medicolegal work. It was abundantly clear how much the US' social security disability, Workers' Compensation and personal injury systems could benefit from incorporating a multidisciplinary approach in assessment of disability and in treatment recommendations.

In the late 1970s, I was fortunate to join the International Association of Study of Pain, the American Pain Society and one of its branches where I resided, the

© Springer International Publishing Switzerland 2015
S. Vasudevan, *Multidisciplinary Management of Chronic Pain*,
DOI 10.1007/978-3-319-20322-5_6

Midwest Pain Society. This was during the "golden age" of chronic pain management when multidisciplinary treatment prevailed. Through active participation in these organizations, I had the opportunity to work closely with notable scientists and "super specialists" including Dr. Dennis Turk, Dr. Richard Chapman, Dr. Wilbert Fordyce, Stephen Brena, M.D. and John Loeser, M.D. These leaders in the pain field, further convinced me that painrelated disability is indeed a treatable problem using the rehabilitation principles I had learned as a physiatrist.

In 1983, the American Academy of Pain Medicine (AAPM), a group composed only of physicians, was formed in the interests of becoming a member group of the American Medical Association (AMA), considered the "voice of medicine" in the United States. While involved with the AAPM, I had the opportunity to serve as President. The AAPM also created the American Board of Pain Medicine (ABPM), to provide certification of physicians who had board certification in other specialties such as Anesthesiology, Neurology, Neurosurgery, Physical Medicine & Rehabilitation (PM&R or Physiatry), Internal Medicine, Family Practice, etc. I was fortunate to be the first and founding President of ABPM, which instituted a certification process for physicians treating individuals with pain.

Although the initial goal was to develop a distinct specialty of Pain Medicine recognized by the American Board of Medical Specialties (ABMS) similar to orthopedic surgery, anesthesiology or neurosurgery, we have yet to see success. However, the ABMS did succeed in interesting the American Board of Anesthesiology (ABA) in establishing a subspecialty in Pain Management/Pain Medicine in the late 1990s.

By 2000, the American Board of Anesthesiology allowed board-certified physicians from the Boards of PM&R and Neurology/Psychiatry to achieve certification in the new subspecialty through taking exams offered by the ABA. By the time this opportunity had arisen, I had personally already gained lifetime Board certification in PM&R in 1978, and by the American Board of Pain Medicine in 1991. I also received the ABA's Certificate of Added Qualification in Pain Medicine and have received 10-year certifications from the American Board of PM&R in the subspeciality of Pain Medicine from 2000 to 2010 and from 2010 to 2020. I also have a lifetime certification from the American Board of Electrodiagnostic Medicine which began in 1979.

Medical professionals who see patients with chronic pain certainly realize that the medical profession is long overdue in recognizing pain as a specialty: as the Institute of Medicine notes, of the 27 institutes in the National Institutes of Health (NIH) not one is dedicated to pain!

Since 1977, I have served as the Medical Director of the multidisciplinary pain clinic at the Curative Rehabilitation center which is part of the Medical College of Wisconsin in Milwaukee. From 1984 to 2000, I served as the Medical Director of a comprehensive pain rehabilitation program at Elmbrook Memorial hospital in Brookfield, Wisconsin. I also directed the Center for Pain and Work Rehabilitation at St. Nicholas Hospital in Sheboygan, Wisconsin, from the early 1990s until 2013.

Since 1994 to the writing of this book in 2015, I have served as Medical Director of the Center for Pain Rehabilitation at Community Memorial Hospital in Menomonee Falls, Wisconsin. I provide care and medical direction for the Center's multidisciplinary treatment, focusing on biopsychosocial and rehabilitation approaches with the goal of improving function and returning patients to work, where possible, while trying to reduce pain. The program, located at the North Hills Health Center, is a joint venture between Community Memorial and Froedtert hospitals and physicians from the Medical College of Wisconsin Community Physicians group.

Everything I share in this book results from my work with such programs which treat the "whole patient" through welcoming families to participate in conferences and treatment meetings and empowering patients through helping them educate themselves about pain.

On the basis of these comprehensive multidisciplinary programs, which I have been privileged to work with since 1977, I sincerely wish that new medical school graduates would be taught to appreciate the psychological, social, cultural, vocational, and environmental factors that may add to or accentuate patients' biological symptoms of pain.

Instead of multiple injections, interventions and repeated surgeries to eliminate or decrease the pain, future physicians can empower their patients through education and enlisting them in their own treatments in shared decision making. In addition to greatly improving the quality of life for chronic pain patients, eliminating excessive expenditures for uncoordinated pain treatments would make a huge difference in healthcare costs.

Multidisciplinary pain rehabilitation "shifts the focus from searching for the pain source, which may not even be identifiable on a test, to what.. .[a patient] can do to become more functional," writes David Hanscom, M.D. (2012). Multidisciplinary treatment "addresses all the factors contributing to chronic pain and a turbo-charged nervous systems—lack of sleep, anxiety, medications, goal setting, physical conditioning, and anger—and goes through the best way to deal with them one by one."

"If you don't stand for something, you will fall for everything"

Patients need to know their choices and the details of the treatments offered before consenting to passive, irreversible treatments such as surgery, stimulators, morphine pumps, and other invasive procedures.

Recently, I came across an editorial in a medical journal that lamented how an "increase in the number of patients per physician" had created the "busy doctor" always attending to "something more urgent than the immediate situation" (James 1974). Patients who were polled for the article saw physicians lacking in time, warmth, and "real" concern for them. The irony is, the editorial was written in 1974, more than 40 years before the writing of this book! Certainly, because of increasing patient loads today and reimbursement patterns, it is easier to offer a patient unimodal and often expensive treatments for chronic pain than our time and listening ear.

> Unless the psychological and social factors behind chronic pain are addressed, physical *rehabilitation, pharmacotherapy and interventional approaches in isolation will be inadequate to treat the multiple needs of patients with chronic pain.*
>
> Sridhar Vasudevan, M.D.

Fundamentals in Treating Pain Patients

Reeducation

By the time we see most pain patients they have internalized some myths about their pain, either from their own unsuccessful course of treatments or simply from living in a society that greatly misunderstands chronic pain. Many of these myths are found in *Treat Your Own Back*, a helpful book for pain patients, the main points of which are shown in Table 6.1 (McKenzie 1980).

Helping the Patient Reframe His Pain

In over 37 years of treating chronic pain patients, I have become convinced that, unless the psychological and social factors behind chronic pain are addressed, *physical rehabilitation, pharmacotherapy and interventional approaches will be*

Table 6.1 Eight myths of back pain adapted from *Treat Your Own Back*

Myth	Truth
Back pain is short-term	For at least half of patients, it is recurrent
Spinal manipulation gives the best results	Gives limited benefits, encourages patient passivity
Ultrasound/electrical therapies are helpful	No long-term benefit, healing not accelerated; underlying problem not addressed
Inflammation causes back pain	Inflammation may accompany some conditions like rheumatoid arthritis but most are entirely mechanical in nature
Pain comes from "degeneration of the spine"	Changes shown on X-rays are rarely pain generators
Pain requires rest	After 1 or 2 days, mobility should be regained
Stop sports like jogging or golf	Patients can likely return to their sports as they recover
Weather causes the pain	Damp conditions and drafts are not behind back pain

inadequate. If the biopsychosocial factors are not included in chronic pain treatment, patients often end up with pain conditions that are characterized by dysfunction, disuse, dramatic pain behaviors, drug misuse/abuse, and disability that far exceed the physical findings.

Then and now I see many patients presenting with failed back surgery syndrome (FBSS), fibromyalgia, complex regional pain syndrome, headaches, neck and extremity pain, and other stubborn conditions in which pain has been firmly established. Many have become discouraged and started to think of themselves as disabled. Yet, almost all of these patients, if they alter their attitude toward their pain and situation—"reframing" their pain—and become open-minded to multidisciplinary treatment, improve. We regularly see them achieve independence, new psychological skills, gain control of their pain and their life, and find alternative work that is compatible with their physical and medical restrictions. They achieve self-responsibility and self-efficacy in the management of their pain and a positive, long-term outcome.

Multidisciplinary Pain Rehabilitation Replaces Negative "CDs" Playing in the Patient's Head

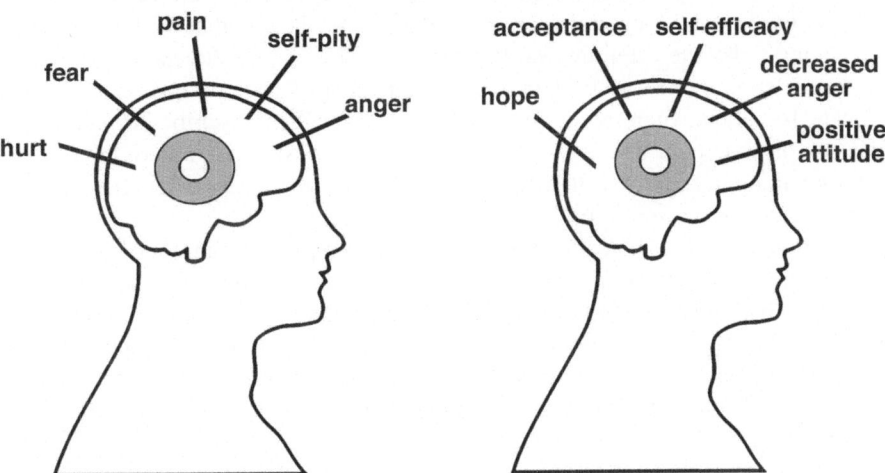

To usher along this transformation, I suggest observing these rules at all times in your treatment of pain patients as shown in Table 6.2.

Rule 1: Pain Is Real

I never question the existence of a patient's pain. In my decades of pain medicine experience, I have applied the rule that I would not judge the existence of someone's pain but would judge the underlying cause, if it can be found, and consider the appropriate combination of treatment to address the "person and the pain." As

Table 6.2 Four rules for clinicians to observe when treating patients with chronic pain

Pain Is Always Real
Pain Is *Always* in the Brain
Inform About Choices
Search Your Own Soul

medical professionals, it is our responsibility to first rule out significant, treatable or correctable pathologies contributing to the pain condition, while not conceding to inappropriate demands for test or treatment. *Then, if there is no clear curable disease/pathology, our focus should be on the person experiencing the pain and not the pain itself.*

Rule 2: Pain Is *Always* in the Brain

We know from the main theories of pain presented in Chap. 3, that the brain modulates almost all pain responses. This is one reason Cognitive Behavioral Therapy techniques and relaxation methods, explained in Chap. 4, and some antidepressants and antiseizure drugs are effective in chronic pain. *It certainly does not mean the pain is "imaginary."* I am surprised and saddened by the fact that medical students graduating today are often unaware of the Gate Theory and the chemical, behavioral, and learning theories of pain described in Chap. 3, including Loeser's Model of pain. Too often, when recent graduates listen to a patient describe his pain or see him demonstrate pain behaviors, they assume there must be an underlying disease or tissue injury in keeping with the Door Bell Theory which says when there is pain, there is a pain generator at the "door."

Unfortunately this biomedical and unimodal perspective can and does lead to seeking the "pain generator" in diagnostic imaging and to physicians and surgeons "reading" the X-ray not the patient. The "X-ray diagnosis," as I sometimes term it, omits consideration of a patient's social, psychological, vocational, legal, cultural, and environmental milieu. It often leads to numerous interventional techniques, though there is little evidence that multiple injections and long-term use of opioids actually lessen pain.

Rule 3: Inform Patients About Their Choices

There is an alternative to the uncoordinated unimodal care most patients have received by the time we see them—multidisciplinary care. Our first responsibility to patients is to avoid harm including the harm of giving them limited information or clarifications about treatments they have been receiving, especially interventions and excessive drug use. *The "new road" of pain management requires more self-responsibility, learning, effort, and participation than most patients expect or want.* The current healthcare system encourages patient passivity, especially when it comes to chronic pain, and patients have understandably adjusted to the role.

When I see new pain patients, I make it clear that there is an alternative road to the chronic opioid therapy, disability, injections, multiple surgeries, and feelings of hopelessness they have endured. While they may not return to their condition prior to their injury or illness, if patients are willing to learn new skills such as appropriate exercises and body movements from physical and occupational therapists and Cognitive Behavioral techniques from psychologists their pain can be managed and they can have a high quality of life. The basics of the biopsychosocial approach, which have been effective through centuries and practiced all over the world, have been and will always be the mainstay in managing chronic pain as well as other chronic illnesses.

Rule 4: Search Your Own Soul

It never hurts for you to apply what my colleague jokingly refers to as the *"your mama test"* with your pain patients—would I recommend the same test, procedure, medication, surgery, or any other course of treatment for my own mother? Or family?

In addition to always taking a patient's pain seriously, we also need to ask ourselves if our practice changes significantly depending on the patient's insurance carrier. Physicians often treat patients with generous insurance coverage such as Workers' Compensation with more tests or diagnostic procedures than patients with limited or no coverage. This may be realistic, based on "covered services" but our philosophy of treatment should be consistent *regardless of insurance coverage or payor source.*

Finally, when it comes to disability, we need to ask ourselves if we understand the long-term implications of recommending a permanent disability rating on patients. Clearly, some patients with injuries or illness, despite optimal treatment, may have to be restricted permanently from certain activities to prevent them from harming themselves or aggravating, precipitating or accelerating an underlying condition. But permanent restrictions, in addition to affecting a patient's future employment and insurance status, also lead to iatrogenic disability. These important issues are explored further in Chap. 7, Evaluation of Disability in Patients with Chronic Pain.

In Chaps. 1, 2, 3, 4, we explored the tremendous effect a patient's belief system, cultural and social milieu, and psychological makeup have on his experience of pain. Several theories suggest the extent to which a patient expresses pain behaviors and feels stress, anger or resentment exert a significant influence on pain. It should be good news to medical professionals seeing chronic pain patients, then, that regardless of the type of pain they present or their particular set of biopsychosocio circumstances, the treatment goals for most chronic pain patients remain remarkably similar!

Our goals are to induce in the patient a sense of self-efficacy and self-responsibility and empower him as a partner in his own pain management through multidisciplinary care, as shown in Table 6.3. This process usually begins with elimination of narcotics and identification of appropriate medication, increasing physical activity, addressing the patient's psychological and emotional issues and educating the patient about pain and pain management.

Table 6.3 Six goals for treating the patient with chronic pain

Eliminate all nonessential medications, especially opioids
Improve sleep patterns and control depression
Increase physical activity, flexibility and endurance; functional improvement is the goal
Improve coping skills through psychological support; encourage self-efficacy
Improve socialization and recreational activities with friends and family
Return patient to work if he is able, even if a different job than before if retired improve quality of life

Multidisciplinary pain rehabilitation offers a patient a "cafeteria" of treatments from stretching and strengthening exercises to physical modalities like heat and Transcutaneous Electrical Nerve Stimulation units (TENS) to psychological tools like Cognitive Behavioral Therapy. To improve a patient's function, control disability and decrease his dependence on the healthcare system, all avenues of pain management should be explored including drugs, injections, and surgeries when appropriate.

An astounding 30–50 % of patients are abusing medications by the time we see them which is why eliminating all nonessential medication is an early and continuing goal. Whether these medications are opioids like oxycodone and hydrocodone, benzodiazepines like Xanax or other habit forming drugs, assessing the patient's current drug use and titrating him off nonessential drugs should be addressed as soon as possible.

If patients have become habituated to opioids, benzodiazepines or related drugs, they usually have a firm conviction that their pain will worsen if they are titrated off the medications and will resist such a plan. Except in rare instances, long-term use of such drugs worsens chronic pain. Many patients share that, contrary to their expectations, their pain actually subsided when they titrated off opioids. The services of an addictionologist are often useful as you help the patient titrate off nonessential medicine.

While, methadone maintenance is often used to reduce or eliminate prescribed opioids, followed by self-monitored abstinence, buprenorphine replacement therapy is gaining hold in helping addicted patients (Ruetsch 2014). Studies suggest "that the commonly used 6-month (minimum) maintenance period for treating opioid abuse may be compressed to 2 weeks of buprenorphine stabilization."

Patients bedeviled with fear of pain who avoid activities they worry will bring pain and display many pain behaviors like sighing, limping and grimacing will largely have to accept your suggestion that opioids are not helping their pain and may be making it worse on faith. Elsewhere in this book, we have likened a pain patient's willingness to try a new and different treatment path as similar to an alcoholic taking the first step in the Twelve Steps of Alcoholics Anonymous. Like pain patients, problem drinkers believe they "need" the alcohol and that it is the answer to their problems—and it may well have been, at one time. But when the drinker is ready to try a new path of treatment, he will admit that the substance that once *helped* him with his problems has *become* his problem. A similar "Gestalt" happens with patients who have become habituated to opioids.

Table 6.4 Nondrug treatments for pain

Education
Exercises
Heat/cold
TENS
Traction
Orthotics
Massage
Manipulation
Relaxation methods
Biofeedback
Cognitive Behavioral
Herbal medicine
Acupuncture
Homeopathy
Spiritual/faith
Family Therapy

In this chapter, we will look at helpful medications that can be used in chronic pain but there are also many *non-pharmacological* treatments which should be tried from hot/cold and TENS units to complementary and alternative medicine (CAM) techniques, as shown in Table 6.4.

Titrating patients off nonessential medication is one of the first ways in which multidisciplinary rehabilitation differs from the contemporary, non-EBM pain treatments we reviewed in Chap. 5. Whereas most chronic pain patients have sought a "cure" or "quick fix," this is the point where the patient must accept that his pain will, in all probability, never completely go away—though, importantly, it can be managed. Whereas the patient has likely received treatments passively, this is the point where he is called on to become an active part of his treatment—physically, through exercises and psychologically through receiving support from health psychologists or social workers and letting go of his negative emotions.

The patient is asked to exert more effort than he has probably had to harness until now and change his entire attitude. He is asked to "check his skepticism and pessimism at the door," though they may have been constant companions he has lived with for years, especially if he has sustained an injury or accident.

I don't think any patient wants to hear from a medical professional that the source of his pain can't be determined and that the pain cannot be cured. Yet, this is the point where both the patient and the physician concur that the patients have had enough surgery and drugs and it is time for a new path. The apparent "bad news" leads to good news. I have thousands of patients who, having accepted that reality and altered their attitude, now say "I was in a car accident" or "I have fibromyalgia" but "I am able to live with it; the pain does not control me."

In my experience, the patients who achieve the best attitude of accepting their pain and taking responsibility for its management are the ones who have learned the difference between "hurt and harm," and been acquainted with the different theories

Table 6.5 Desirable changes in patient outlook

No longer seeking a cure or quick fix
No interest in further surgeries or interventions
Willing to titrate off nonessential drug
Open-mindedness toward new way
Willing to give up passive care and become partner
Willing to do physical and mental "work"—self-efficacy
Willing to give up anger, pessimism, and self-pity. Reframing; Cognitive Behavioral, Relaxation therapies

that explain pain as shown in Table 6.5. They have been taught stretching exercises, how to perform their activities of daily living (ADL) without pain and how to avoid dependence on both their medication and the healthcare system itself.

Treating Chronic Pain Patients with Medication

It is not the intention of this book to provide specific dosages or drug regimens for drugs that have proved useful in chronic pain. It is recommended that you refer to valuable sources like *Evaluation and Treatment of Chronic Pain* (Aronoff 1999), the *Physician's Desk Reference* (2011) or an online resource, www.epocrates.com for specific information on the medications discussed here.

In assessing a patient's pain, we need to recognize the difference between nociceptive and neuropathic pain as shown in Table 6.6. Nociceptive pain is a response associated with tissue injury from pathologic process in an intact nervous system, where the intensity of pain is proportionate to the injury, and serves as a protective mechanism for the patient. Neuropathic pain, on the other hand, is due to dysfunction or injury to the nervous system that produces disproportionate pain to the stimulus and does not serve a protective and biologically useful function. The two types of pain are treated differently including the medications that are prescribed. While nociceptive pain responds to both opioids and non-opioid drugs, including nonsteroidal anti-inflammatory drugs (NSAIDs), there is little evidence that NSAIDs provide relief of neuropathic pain, though they may be helpful in combination with other drugs and even topically, which we look at later in this chapter.

In Chap. 5 and elsewhere in this book, I have expressed concerns about the overuse of opioids in chronic pain management. Not only do opioids only provide 20–30 % relief, according to Richard W. Rosenquist, M.D., some patients experience worsening of their pain from opioids, a phenomenon called "opioid-induced hyperalgesia" or OIA (Rosenquist 2014).

"If you give an antibiotic for a UTI and it doesn't treat the infection, you stop it," says Dr. Rosenquist. "The same principle applies [to opioids]. Many patients are on opioids for a long time without ever achieving a good outcome, yet their providers fail to question it and try something different."

In a pain newsletter from the Cleveland Clinic, Dr. Rosenquist also notes how the "pendulum" has swung back about the safety of opioid drugs, as we noted in earlier chapters. In the late 1980s, an effort took hold among pain specialists to improve chronic pain treatment through expanded opioid use, notes Dr. Rosenquist. "Opioids were known to be effective for acute pain, so the thinking was, Why not use them for patients with chronic pain who need greater relief?" Clinicians at the time believed that if the indications were legitimate, patients would not become addicted but "reality caught up with us," says Dr. Rosenquist. "We learned that people who get started on opioids have a much higher conversion to active addiction than previously thought. Also, physical dependence on opioids develops quickly, and in some people it turns into physical addiction."

As the medical profession is increasingly recognizing, there is little evidence of the value of long-term prescription of opioids in relieving chronic pain, disability or helping a patient return to work. In fact, some data show opioid therapy may actually delay a patient's return to the work force. In my experience, opioid treatment for chronic pain has the following drawbacks:

1. It increases patients' beliefs that they have an unusual and significant condition that requires opioid analgesia, thus reinforcing illness behavior and disability conviction.
2. Although opioids do not produce end-organ damage compared with other analgesics, they lead individuals to become dependent on the healthcare system, which can be as problematic—as the physical dependence on opioids.
3. Chronic opioid therapy, while perceived as cheaper, easier, and quicker treatment than implementing pain rehabilitation, prevents patients from taking responsibility and control for the pain and their lives.
4. It keeps patients in the care of physicians who prescribe these medications on a long-term basis who may not be appropriate pain clinicians.
5. It increases the perception within the family that the patient has significant medical illness and family members may continue to reinforce the pain behaviors.
6. It prevents patients from discovering they can function fully without the need or use of opioids.
7. It often induces personality changes in users and noted by some patients, family members and medical professionals such as irritability, depression. These can range from amotivational syndromes to actually antisocial or law-breaking behavior.

Because of these considerations, responsible opioid prescribing includes a careful attention to the five A's as seen in Table 6.6 and documentation.

Table 6.6 Five "A's" to Monitor During Opioid Treatment	
	Analgesia-increased pain relief
	Activities-Increase in function
	Aberrant behavior-monitor and document
	Adverse effects-note and treat
	Affect-Mood—should improve/less depression

1. **Analgesia** pain relief must be provided. On a 10-point scale where 0 is no pain and 10 is unbearable pain, only use opioids if they decrease pain to 3–5 from 7–8.
2. **Activities** must be increasing. Only keep a patient on opioids if he is becoming able to accomplish more activities of daily living, resuming productive work and participating in social activities at higher levels. There needs to be a documented increase in function.
3. **Aberrant** behaviors must not be observed. The patient must not be getting the drug from more than one physician, "losing" prescriptions, getting early refills, escalating doses or failing to use as prescribed. A urine drug test can determine if a patient is taking his drugs or selling or diverting them instead. When prescribed medications are not found or non-prescribed medications or illegal medications *are* found such as cocaine or marijuana, an abnormal urine drug test will be reported. Marijuana is still illegal in many US states.
4. **Adverse** effects must be absent. Side effects like sleepiness, fatigue, constipation, confusion, dizziness and euphoria should not be preventing the patient from improved functioning or ability to drive. Some side effects resolve with time but constipation will persist and stool softeners are always needed for chronic opioid treatment. Opioids also can cause and add to depression and depressed patients should have access to counseling and appropriate antidepressant medications and other mental health resources.
5. **Affect** or patient's mood should be improving. When used in the right doses in the right person, a patient's mood and function will improve with opioid medications. If the person is misusing or abusing opioids, on the other hand, his mood will often worsen. If a patient shows negative mood change and worsening depression, with no improvement in function, he should be taken off opioids or other drugs.

Non-opioid Medication

Luckily, for those of us seeing pain patients, there are other medications which prove very useful in treating chronic pain and often offer better safety profiles than opioids. When treating chronic pain, it is important to decide what type of pain is being treated. Using the wrong treatment for the wrong type of pain will clearly be unsuccessful.

Here is a short synopsis of the types of pain and which treatment would be appropriate, as seen in Table 6.7:

Table 6.7 Types of pain and appropriate treatments

Nociceptive pain	NSAIDs; cautiously opioids
Inflammatory pain	NSAIDs
Mechanical pain	Assistive devices, modifications, manual therapies
Neuropathic pain	Antiseizure drugs, antidepressants, short-term sympathetic blocks
Psychological pain	Psychologist; psychiatrist
Multiple causes of pain	Multidisciplinary treatment

1. Nociceptive pain—If there is still ongoing, clearly identifiable tissue injury, NSAIDs (anti-inflammatory drugs) and some types of opioids, like Tramadol or hydrocodone, used selectively to improve function may be considered.
2. Inflammatory pain—If there is evidence of a flare up of arthritis or muscle injury, a short course of NSAIDs will be beneficial.
3. Mechanical pain—If there is a structural problem such as unhealed bones in the foot and ankle after a fracture or spinal pain due to muscle tightness or local mechanical dysfunction, drugs have no role here. In these situations, physical approaches such as shoe modification, assistive devices like a cane or manual therapies such as myofascial release or a home program, are what is needed.
4. Neuropathic pain—It there is an injury or dysfunction of the nervous system or the sympathetic nervous system, opioids have *not* proved effective. In some conditions, such as complex regional pain syndrome (CRPS), 3–4 sympathetic blocks may decrease sympathetically mediated pain often seen in CRPS patients. The most useful drugs for neuropathic pain are antiseizure and antidepressant drugs, discussed more fully later in this chapter.
5. Psychological pain—Where there are many psychological factors such as depression, anger, catastrophisizing, anticipatory pain, anxiety, illness, and disability conviction with insufficient medical basis for the claimed disability/illness, the psychosocial treatment by a trained psychologist and counselor (with a psychiatrist if needed) should be the emphasis of treatment.
6. Multiple causes—Patients with FBSS fibromyalgia, or work-related or car accident-related chronic pain with numerous biopsychosocial-legal issues need multidisciplinary treatment. Unimodality treatment in such conditions will worsen pain and disability and lead to an added burden on society by increasing healthcare costs with poor outcome.

Prescription Medications

The drug classes used for pain include nonsteroidal anti-inflammatory drugs (NSAIDs), opioids, both tricyclic and SNRI antidepressants, antiseizure drugs (sometimes called antiepileptic drugs (AED), anticonvulsants or neuromodulators), antiarrhythmics, topical formulations and more. These drugs may be combined to produce synergistic effects such as targeting different sites along the neural axis, called "rational polypharmacy." However, combining drugs with similar modes of actions is not recommended.

Nonsteroidal Anti-inflammatory Drugs

Nonsteroidal anti-inflammatory drugs (NSAIDs) such as aspirin, naproxen, and ibuprofen, commonly used to treat arthritic pain, have not proved useful for chronic pain unless used in combination with other drugs. While NSAIDs inhibit both forms of the COX enzyme, COX-1 and COX-2, it is the latter that is responsible for the inflammatory response and pain. COX-1, on the other hand, protects the gastrointestinal system though production of prostaglandin in the gut mucosa and therefore suppression of the COX-1 enzyme carries obvious risks. The introduction of selective COX-2 inhibitors like celecoxib (Celebrex), rofecoxib (Vioxx), and valdecoxib (Bextra) which did not suppress COX-1 was initially greeted as positive news for chronic pain patients. Though rofecoxib (Vioxx) and valdecoxib (Bextra) seemed truly "magical," according to some patients, in treating pain, if they were taken for more than a few weeks they exerted serious cardiovascular effects and were subsequently taken off the market. The only COX-2 inhibitor remaining on the market is celecoxib (Celebrex) which does not seem to block the enzyme which caused the dangerous rofecoxib (Vioxx) and valdecoxib (Bextra) side effects, which included heart attacks and strokes.

NSAIDs should be used cautiously in patients at risk of hypertension and edema and until their risk of induced GI complication is determined. A prophylactic agent such as a proton pump inhibitor or Misoprostol may be added.

Tricyclic Antidepressants

Tricyclic antidepressants such as amitriptyline, imipramine, clomipramine, nortriptyline, desipramine, and maprotiline were the preferred way of treating depression until SSRI antidepressants like Prozac debuted in the late 1980s.

Yet tricyclics also exert neuromodulatory effects on chronic pain and the effects are seen at low doses. For desipramine, nortriptyline, amitriptyline, and imipramine, patients can be given a starting dosage of as low as 10 mg increased by increments. Neuropathic pain responds more quickly than depression to tricyclics and effects in chronic pain patients may be seen in 3–10 days. They are currently the first-line treatment of neuropathic pain, in my practice.

The adverse effects of tricyclics, which are most pronounced in the elderly, are constipation, dry mouth, blurred vision, cognitive changes, tachycardia, urinary hesitation, orthostatic hypotension, falls, weight gain, sedation and notably EKG conduction abnormalities. The secondary amines like desipramine and nortriptyline exhibit fewer anticholinergic and sedative effects than do the tertiary amines like amitriptyline, imipramine, and doxepin are preferable.

Selective Norepinephrine Reuptake Inhibitors

Selective Norepinephrine Reuptake Inhibitor (SNRIs) antidepressants, which have succeeded Selective Serotonin Reuptake Inhibitors (SSRIs) for use in some depressed patients, are also proving useful in the treatment of chronic pain. The identification of these drugs for use in chronic pain stems from growing awareness that norepinephrine is a greater modulator in the pain process than serotonin, and some have been US Food and Drug Administration-approved for neuropathic pain and fibromyalgia. These drugs include venlafaxine (Effexor), duloxetine (Cymbalta), and the newer drugs milnacipran (Savella) and levomilnacipran (Fetzima), the latter being an isomer of milnacipran. An early SNRI, sibutramine, used for the treatment of obesity and sold as Meridia was withdrawn from US markets in 2010 due to risk of serious cardiovascular events (FDA 2010). Duloxetine (Cymbalta) is one of the few drugs approved by the FDA for neuropathic pain and it is the second-choice drug in my practice. It is also approved for fibromyalgia, and certain types of musculoskeletal pain, like osteoarthritis. Milnacipran (Savella) is the other drug currently FDA-approved for fibromyalgia. These drugs also help in a patient's depression, especially Cymbalta which can become psychoactively effective in 2–4 weeks.

While these antidepressants can be useful in chronic pain treatment, they are also associated with side effects and adverse reactions. Duloxetine, which is FDA-approved for neuropathic pain, chronic osteoarthritis pain, chronic low back pain and fibromyalgia, is contraindicated in patients with heavy alcohol use or chronic liver disease, in whom it presents a risk of acute hepatitis. Milnacipran, which is approved for fibromyalgia, carries the risks of serotonin syndrome, elevated blood pressure and heart rate, hepatotoxicity and seizures. Levomilnacipran, not approved for fibromyalgia, carries similar risks along with abnormal bleeding and angle closure glaucoma. All antidepressants carry risk of suicidal ideation so patients need to be carefully monitored.

Antiseizure Drugs

Antiseizure drugs have proved a bright spot in the pharmacological treatment of chronic pain. One reason for the recruitment of such drugs in pain management is that the "gate" postulated in the Gate and the Neuromatrix theories, is now regarded to be a *chemical gate* rather than an *electrical* gate consisting of just nerve conduction. Even when Melzack and Wall originally advanced their Gate Theory in 1965, which postulated that the body had a mechanism that could "open" and "close" pain perception, some scientists sought to understand better what bioevents actually "operate the gate." Allan Basbaum, Ph.D., now professor at the UCSF School of Medicine, and other scientists undertook research which led to a better understanding of chemical mediators like prostaglandin, substance P, aldolase, glutamate, serotonin, norepinephrine, endorphin, and GABA on pain. Their discoveries, in turn, led to the increasing use of antidepressants and antiseizure drugs in pain management.

Before our understanding of their actions, antiseizure drugs were used for over 30 years on an empirical or experimental basis to control pain, especially when the cause was not clear. In fact, the abnormal processing of visual and other sensations seen in syndromes like fibromyalgia, sometimes called "sensory amplification," is similar to the nerves having a "seizure." Some researchers now believe these nerves

Table 6.8 Main antiseizure drugs

First generation, older	Second generation, newer
Phenytoin	Gabapentin/pregabalin
Phenobarbital	Topiramate
Primidone	Lamotrigine
Ethosuximide	Tiagabine
Carbamazepine	Levetiracetam
Valproic acid	Zonisamide

appear to "seize" because the messages of neurotransmitters like serotonin and dopamine are not received and these medications modulate the chemical messages received via ion channels. When patients have nerve damage after surgery that is persistent or burning or when patients are under emotional stress, these chemically modulating medications can be particularly effective.

The action of the first generation anticonvulsants, such as gabapentin (Neurontin) is believed to stem from their interaction with voltage-gated Ca^{2+} channels thought to dampen seizure activity. The drugs also reduce pain-related responses after peripheral inflammation and reduce or prevent allodynia and hyperalgesia. Second-generation anticonvulsants such as pregabalin (Lyrica) are thought to exert effects on the Alpha2-delta ligand, binding at voltage-gated calcium channels and causing their analgesic, anxiolytic, and anticonvulsant activity. Lyrica has been approved for neuropathic pain and fibromylgia. It is the third-line drug in my practice. The main antiseizure drugs are shown in Table 6.8.

Side effects to be expected with the use of first generation antiseizure drugs include drowsiness and lethargy as several of the drugs are molecularly related to barbiturates. Second generation antiseizure drugs like gabapentin and pregabalin can also cause sleepiness as well as dizziness, weight gain, swelling of the hands and feet, dry mouth and suicidal thoughts or behavior.

Several other antiseizure drugs, lamotrigine, zonisamide, levetiracetam and tiagabine, have been empirically used, although they are *not* approved for neuropathic pain. They should be prescribed with caution as they carry warnings for Stevens-Johnson syndrome and toxic epidermal necrolysis, potentially lethal side effects, which clearly limit their usefulness. Warnings that accompany topiramate, which is approved for the treatment of migraine headaches, should also be noted. They include suicidal thoughts or behavior, visual problems, metabolic disorders, cognitive dysfunction and fetal toxicity.

Other Oral Medications

Other oral medications used in chronic pain treatment include clonidine, a centrally acting alpha-agonist hypotensive agent that decreases heart rate and relaxes the blood vessels, and tramadol, a centrally acting atypical opioid analgesic which also blocks serotonin and norepinephrine reuptake. Many patients respond well to tramadol whose soporific effects are helpful in inducing sleep. Some of tramadol's pain reduction actions stem from its mixture of both R- and S-stereoisomers, which are thought to complement each other's analgesic activity.

Other drugs seen in chronic pain treatment include corticosteroids such as prednisone which are useful when inflammation is present and N-methyl-D-aspartate receptor (NMDAR) antagonist drugs like ketamine and dextromethorphan. The rationale for NMDAR antagonist drugs stems from the effect of increased NMDAR activity on central sensitization in certain types of neuropathic pain. There are other treatments that researchers are currently investigating including aldose reductase inhibitors, neurotropic factors, vascular endothelial growth factor, gamma linolenic acid, protein kinase C beta inhibitors, immune therapy, hyperbaric oxygen and alpha lipoic acid.

Topical Medications

Topical medications serve as the "workhorse" of much chronic pain treatment because of their direct access to the site of pain, avoidance of first-pass metabolism, patient adherence and acceptance and, of course, their lack of side effects when compared to oral medications.

The 5 % lidocaine patch (Lidoderm patch) was the first medication approved for pain after shingles. It is approved and used for variety of neuropathic pain conditions, with varying results. It has been empirically found to be useful in treating lower back pain, myofascial pain syndrome, complex regional pain syndrome, osteoarthritis, and a variety of neuropathic pain and musculoskeletal conditions. The lack of side effects associated with the lidocaine patch makes it an appropriate option for any focal neuropathic pain with allodynia or hyperalgesia (Zempsky 2013).

Topical NSAIDS, as shown in Table 6.9, are used effectively in some pain conditions such as osteoarthritis and acute musculoskeletal injury. NSAIDs when used topically are not linked to the increased bleeding seen with oral use and their risk of gastrointestinal side effects is much lower yet they achieve 4–7 times the levels in muscular tissues of an oral dose.

Capsaicin, derived from chili peppers, is considered a "counter-irritant" which attenuates the sensation of pain by acting as an irritant on a painful zone. Capsaicin is a TRPV1 agonist which exerts two actions: first it activates nociceptive nerve

Table 6.9 Main agents found in topical treatments	
	Lidocaine
	NSAIDs
	Capsaicin
	Methyl salicylates
	menthol
	Dexamethasone
	Arnica

Table 6.10 Exercise should
include

Range of motion
Flexibility
Muscle strengthening
Aerobic conditioning

fibers in the skin engendering the release of substance P, which results in neurogenic inflammation. This is followed by "reversible defunctionalization of nerve endings resulting in the inhibition of pain transmission," explains William Zempsky, M.D. Other counter-irritants used as topical treatments are methyl salicylates, which warm tissue through vasodilatory effects in addition to analgesia and menthol which cools the skin. Other topically used drugs are dexamethasone, a steroid which can treat inflammatory conditions, the perennial herb arnica, the spasticity drug baclofen, gamma-aminobutyric acid (GABA), nitrates, and even tricyclic antidepressants. Cooling sprays such as Biofreeze are also available and useful.

When pharmacotherapy is used, prescribers should consider efficacy, adverse side effects, dosing frequency, patient preference, and cost in selecting medications. Make sure to educate your patients about the medications being prescribed.

Pharmacotherapy is, of course, only one part of multidisciplinary treatment and should be used in conjunction with nutritional, physical, educational, and cognitive behavioral treatments. Patients should receive information from the clinicians treating their pain about anatomy, self-help techniques, and physical modalities (including heat/cold application exercise), relaxation, good nutritional habits, coping with painful activities and other pain management techniques.

Weight management should be an integral part of patient education, especially increasing the patient's awareness of the relationship between healthy body weight and pain. Physical activity is a basic part of treatment and patients should participate in moderate-intensity physical activity at least 3–4 times a week that includes range of motion, flexibility, muscle strengthening, and aerobic conditioning exercises. If patients are at risk for cardiovascular events, they should be instructed to take a daily, low-dose of aspirin (81 mg) unless otherwise indicated. The ideal exercises for pain patients are shown in Table 6.10.

If patients lack resources or motivation to exercise, they can explore group classes in the community which can add impetus, serve a social function, and are often free of charge. Patients can also be referred to physical or exercise therapists.

Elderly Patients

Most chronic pain conditions are found in elderly patients, yet medication and treatment guidelines are often written with the younger patient in mind. Therefore it is important to observe the following in the management of your older patients' pain, as seen in Tables 6.11 and 6.12 (Makris et al. 2014).

Table 6.11 Overview for elderly patient care	Determine comorbidities, cognitive and functional status and social/family circumstances
	Use multidisciplinary approach with drug/nondrug treatment; physical/occupational therapy
	Ascertain if patient has a reliable physician who responds promptly to calls and provides backup
	Be willing to revisit previously used modalities with modifications as needed
	Involve caregivers and seek out resources in community as needed
	Reinforce progress and give patient encouragement at each visit

Table 6.12 Overview for pharmacology in elderly patient care	Explain the medications in terms of benefits in daily living and functioning
	Use medications that enhance each other's pain reduction when possible
	Acetaminophen should be first-line for mild-to-moderate pain
	Avoid long-term oral NSAIDs due to cardiovascular, gastrointestinal, and other effects
	Opioids may be tried if no response to first-line drugs with caution
	Consider SSRI or SNRIs in patients with depression
	Monitor patients for efficacy, tolerability, and adherence with new treatments
	Encourage physical activity including physical therapy and exercise
	Connect patients with Cognitive Behavioral and movement therapy resources
	Monitor patients for goal achievement, modify treatment as needed

Medication Is Only Part of Multidisciplinary Care

If you educate your patient in the many factors behind pain and instill in him a new willingness, open-mindedness and dedication to practice self-management and self-efficacy in his pain, you will likely be very pleased with the outcome. A good way to approach care for the chronic pain patient is to remember the precepts in "I Am Special."

I is for information regarding pain, including the Gate and Door Bell Theories, medications, and other issues related to chronic pain.

A is for alternatives for treatment, including medical, physical, psychological, psychiatric, and complementary and alternative care.

Table 6.13 Main points of this chapter

Clinicians must appreciate many factors behind pain
Respect a patient's pain
Cultivate a new attitude in patient
Educate the patient about options
Discourage opioid treatment
Explore non-opioid treatments
Use a breadth of modalities
Encourage self-management and self-efficacy

M is for medications and the importance of taking proper drugs in their proper amounts for the right time and for the right purpose.

S is for surgical treatment which the patient should discuss with a surgeon, if necessary.

P is for physical exercise and pacing activities.

E is for emotion. Increased anger, anxiety, and frustration increase pain and Cognitive Behavioral therapies can reduce.

C is for pain clinics and counseling, important tools in pain management.

I is for insight and the patient **I**ncorporating his newly acquired knowledge into his day-to-day activities.

A is for activities and the importance of the patient staying active and avoiding deconditioning.

L is for living a productive and functional life without dependency on the healthcare system, medication or others.

More clinical guidance on the multidisciplinary treatment of chronic pain including case studies appear in Chap. 7, Evaluation of Disability in Patients with Chronic Pain and in Chap. 8, Creating a Multidisciplinary Team.

References

Aronoff, G. (1999). *Evaluation and treatment of chronic pain.* New York: Lippincott Williams & Wilkins.

FETZIMA. (2014). Highlights of prescribing information. Forest Laboratories.

Hanscom, D. (2012). *Back in control.* Seattle, WA: Vertus Press.

Institute of Medicine. (2011). *Relieving pain in America* (p. 11). Washington, DC: National Academy of Sciences.

James, T. (1974). The busy doctor stereotype. *Wisconsin Medical Journal, 113*(4), 129–130.

Food and Drug Administration (2014). Living with fibromyalgia, drugs approved to manage pain.

Lyrica. (2014). Highlights of prescribing information. Pfizer.

Makris, E., Abrams, R., & Gurland, B. (2014). Management of persistent pain in the older patient. *Journal of the American Medical Association, 312*(8), 825–838.

McCleane, G. (2003). Topical use of nitrates, capsaicin and tricyclic antidepressants for pain management. *Advanced Studies in Medicine, 3*, S631–S634.

McKenzie, R. (1980). *Treat your own back* (9th ed., pp. 5–9). Minneapolis, MN: OPTP.

Meridia (sibutramine): Market Withdrawal Due to Risk of Serious Cardiovascular Events. (2010). Food and Drug Administration. Retrieved from http://www.fda.gov/safety/medwatch/safetyinformation/safetyalertsforhumanmedicalproducts/ucm228830.htm

Physicians' Desk Reference (2011). 66th ed. Montvale, NJ: PDR Network.

Prednisone. (2014). Wikipedia. Retrieved from http://en.wikipedia.org/wiki/Prednisone

Rosenquist, R. (2014). A hard lesson learned over two decades: Why specialists rarely use opioids for chronic pain. *Pain Consult*. Cleveland Clinic.

Ruetsch, C. (2014). Treating prescription opioid dependence. *Journal of the American Medical Association, 312*(11), 1145–1146.

Savella. (2013). Highlights of prescribing information. Forest Laboratories.

Topamax. (2009). Highlights of prescribing information. Janssen Pharmaceuticals.

Tramadol. (2014).Wikipedia. Retrieved from http://en.wikipedia.org/wiki/Tramadol

Zempsky, W. (2013, September). Use of topical analgesics in treating neuropathic and musculo-skeletal pain. *Pain Medicine News*.

Zonegran. (2004). Highlights of prescribing information. Eisai.

Chapter 7
Evaluation of Disability in Patients with Chronic Pain

Any clinician who sees patients with pain will likely see patients with disabilities. Because claims of disability affect the workplace, through federal and private insurance programs and injury litigation, these patients and their cases can be complicated, time consuming, and frustrating. This chapter will provide you an overview of the issues involved in disability-related medicine so you can guide and support your patients. Even though disability medicine often involves monetary payments, case workers, and insurers, the same multidisciplinary pain treatment concepts apply as they do to other chronic pain conditions.

There is no clear correlation between pain and disability, as we have noted in previous chapters nor is there much correlation between relief from pain and greater functionality and return to work (Meier 2013). Moreover, pain linked to work-related and motor vehicle injuries is among the hardest to treat due to the hidden and overt effects of anger, resentment and feelings of being a "victim," medicolegal factors and family involvement. Complicating the situation are medical, legal, and financial systems that reinforce a disability conviction for patients, insurers, and even clinicians who add inadvertently to the problem by using single modality approaches like opioids, surgery, and injections in isolation and without a supporting multidisciplinary pain approach. As in almost all chronic pain conditions, multidisciplinary pain rehabilitation has an excellent track record when treating disability.

In his eye-opening book, *Worried Sick* (2008), Nortin Hadler, M.D. observes the philosophical paradox of workers trying to get well in a disability system that forces them to prove they are "ill." Similarly, many researchers have questioned whether disability programs like the US Workers' Compensation system discourage or slow patients' return to work. Burns et al. found, in their research, "support for the popular notion that patients receiving WC [Workers' Compensation] report more symptoms of pain and greater disability…and may respond less well to treatment than non-WC patients" and cite "pessimistic perception of their ability to return to their

© Springer International Publishing Switzerland 2015
S. Vasudevan, *Multidisciplinary Management of Chronic Pain*,
DOI 10.1007/978-3-319-20322-5_7

former jobs" as a significant factor in nonreturn to work. Other researchers cite the terms "compensation neurosis," "compensation disease" or "accident/litigation neurosis" to explain patients' slow recovery and embracing of a disability conviction, often seen in disability systems (Burns et al. 2005).

But Dworkin et al., while they agree that "compensation benefits" predict "poorer short-term outcomes," suggest the poor outcomes are largely explained by the simple fact that these patients are "less likely to be working" (Dworkin et al. 1985). Moreover, the researchers speculate that "Greater emphasis on patient education, counseling, and vocational intervention," features of multidisciplinary treatment, are positive factors in worker outcomes that are not always quantified or considered when evaluating return to work rates.

And, there are other paradoxes in contemporary disability medicine. Despite our greater understanding of the biochemical and biopsychosocial processes behind chronic pain and the replacement of many physical jobs with desk jobs in the United States and other industrialized countries, low back pain is still "the most common cause of job-related disability" says the National Institute of Neurological Disorders and Stroke (2014).

The psychological goals of multidisciplinary treatment for chronic pain patients in general—a reduction in illness behaviors, catastrophizing and fear avoidance and an increase in positive self-talk, self-efficacy, and self-care (found in Chaps. 1–4 of this book)—are, not surprisingly, associated with positive outcomes in injured workers (Tait 2013). Tait uses the term "presenteeism" to describe the coping skills needed for patients to maintain ongoing employment in the face of chronic pain. The skillset includes positive self-talk, task persistence, less belief in a "medical cure," less need for "tangible support" and a high capacity to ignore or control pain, as we see in Table 7.1.

Yet, since the 1990s, expensive and uncoordinated treatments like surgery and opioids have supplanted multidisciplinary care under the erroneous view of cost-effectiveness, though outcomes suggest otherwise (Meier 2013). For example, Rogers found that multidisciplinary care such as work hardening/work conditioning was more cost-effective in disability cases than surgery. Lower back pain patients

Table 7.1 Predictors of positive disability outcomes in workers	
Positive self-talk
Task persistence
No expectation of "cure"—focus on control
Self-care and self-support
Ability to ignore or control pain
Minimal catastrophizing
Minimal fear avoidance and guarding
Minimal dependency on healthcare system
Little or no opioid medication

who received work hardening/work conditioning but not surgery were half as likely to go on to have surgery and had five times fewer physician visits than those who had surgery but no work hardening/work conditioning, according to insurance information (Rogers et al. 2013). For this reason, even though work hardening/work conditioning can initially increase medical costs from $3000 to $9000, the programs actually save about $1600 per patient when lost wages and reinjury costs are factored in.

Surgery and Opioids Not Cost-Effective Over Time

Lumbar fusion surgery is popular in the Workers' Compensation system but outcomes are anything but positive. Two years after lumbar fusion surgery, 26 % of workers had returned to work versus 67 % of workers who did not have fusion surgery (Nguyen et al. 2010). After the surgery, 27 % of the surgery patients needed reoperations and 36 % had complications. Eleven percent of the surgical patients became permanently disabled versus 2 % of the nonsurgical patients. Patients who had surgery missed, on the average, 1140 work days versus nonsurgical patients who missed an average of 316 days (Nguyen et al. 2010). As we noted in Chaps. 1–5, many popular medical procedures for pain lack evidence-base and justifications for their added expense.

While lumbar spine fusion has positive outcomes with spondylolisthesis with instability, traumatic fracture, and tumors, surgery for other diagnoses remain controversial (Nguyen et al. 2010). Nevertheless, 84 % of the studied Workers' Compensation patients had lumbar spine fusion for disk degeneration, disk herniation, and radiculopathy.

Lumbar surgery also drove opioid use (Nguyen et al. 2010). After lumbar fusion surgery, the use of opioid medications went up by 41 % of patients and 76 % of patients in the Workers' Compensation system who were studied remained on opioids.

An average Workers' Compensation claim without opioids was reported in 2012 to be $13,000 but when short-acting opioids like Percocet are added, it leaps to $39,000. Add *long-acting* opioids like OxyContin and the figure skyrockets to $117,000. An analysis by Accidental Fund Holdings concluded that a workplace injury costs nine times more when treated with opioids. Both private and public employees like firefighters and police officers are excessively treated with long-term opioids with the latter's costs borne by taxpayers (Meier 2013).

A 2008 study in the journal *Spine* found people kept on opioids for more than 7 days during the first 6 weeks after an injury were more than twice as likely to be disabled and out of work a year later (Fauber 2012). A study of 300,000 Workers' Compensation claims by the Workers' Compensation Research Institute found pain and day-to-day function do not improve in workers when they stay on opioids (Meier 2013). In 2009, the US Centers of Disease Control and Prevention noted that opioids are involved in 14,800 overdose deaths a year (Ranavaya 2012).

Factors Which Complicate Disability

Patients with disability, especially when associated with pain, require you to understand the multidimensional nature of the pain phenomenon, as we discussed in Chaps. 1–5. You also need a basic understanding of the different definitions of disability in their medical and legal contexts to determine residual functional abilities and help the patient return to work.

When you have patients with chronic pain presenting for disability evaluations, the use of opioids complicates your job because many of these patients have an associated dependency on opioids. As we have noted in previous chapters, the harmful effects of opioid abuse include hyperalgesia, endocrine problems, sleep abnormalities, immune deficiency, and cognitive impairment all of which contribute to the rate of disability (Ranavaya 2012). A high percentage of pain patients also have depressive symptoms or other psychopathology symptoms that preceded their chronic pain complaints and may be "self-medicating" with non-prescribed drugs and alcohol use. It is important to exercise an index of suspicion when evaluating disability in patients with use or dependency on opioids and other addictive drugs.

As medical professionals treating pain, our job is not to doubt patients' pain but to find reasons and treatment for it. However, as we note in Chap. 10 when discussing Complex Regional Pain Syndrome, sometimes patients can exhibit "factitious" conditions—or malingering. While we do not want to be excessively suspicious of patients, including those seeking disability compensation, there are some warning signs that a patient is not totally "above board" such as inconsistencies in his story, "selective" amnesia, alcohol and drug abuse, noncooperation with care and records that show a spotty work history, as seen in Table 7.2 (Jacks 1994).

When treating patients with disabilities or disability claims, we have to navigate a complicated and frustrating system made even more difficult by the prospect of financial awards, adversarial parties and volatile emotions and the frequent lack of correlation between symptoms of pain and associated disability. No wonder, clinicians have sometimes shied away from patients with disability claims or complaints.

Table 7.2 Signs of possible patient symptom exaggeration/magnification

Medical records	Complaints exceed clinical findings
Timing of pain	Symptoms worse as return to work approaches
Inconsistencies	Claims of dysfunction shift
Spotty work history	Fired, long unemployment periods
Selective amnesia	Omitting relevant information
Noncooperation	Missed appointment, imperious attitude
Litigation history	Patient overly legalistic
Personality problems	Antisocial, anti-authority, dishonest
Drug/alcohol abuse	Records show use; patient denies

It is not the purpose of this chapter to provide step-by-step guidelines for performing disability evaluations. Instead, this chapter will give you an overview and conceptual framework for the medical determination of disability and an introduction to the many disability systems in the United States. I am including in this chapter, highlights of a presentation I gave at the 15th World Congress of Pain, a meeting of the International Association for the Study of Pain (IASP), in Buenos Aires, Argentina in 2014.

While I have personally conducted thousands of disability evaluations on patients under my care as well as "independent medical evaluations" for other claimants, I understand that you may prefer to refer patients to physicians or specialists who are experts in evaluating disability, especially in complex personal injuries like car accidents, slip and falls, or medical malpractice which result in injury to a person and possible permanent disability.

Still, we are often asked by attorneys, social security agencies, insurance carriers, and other physicians to provide assessments of patient disabilities including residual functional capacity in patients involved in private short or long-term disability policies, FMLA (Family Medical Leave Act), or short-term time "away from work" or "return to work with restrictions" determinations after a mild, self-limiting work injury. In these cases, it is often important for the primary care provider (MD, DO, NP, or PA) to provide timely information by completing forms patients may bring to their appointment, so that your patients are compensated and can receive the appropriate treatment.

It is also important for you to be fair and objective in these disability evaluations and to remember that society entrusts us with helping to compensate the patient adequately for injuries and illnesses that require time off work. At the end of this chapter, there is a reference list of books that would be helpful, if you wish to understand the disability determination process better.

A Framework for Understanding Disability

Like pain, disability is a highly complex and sometimes subjective medical designation with a variety of interpretations and governed by disparate systems. Historically, social justice systems and the concept of disability can be traced back to medieval times, where the "whole person" concept originated—meaning intactness of the body. Injury that resulted in some loss of body parts or function led to efforts to restore that "whole person" as closely as possible to the person inferred to have existed prior to injury. Laws that compensate workers deemed to be disabled can be traced back to Germany in 1911 which provided assistance in restoring an injured worker to competitive employment (Vasudevan and Ajuwon 2014).

Most people searching through the literature addressing pain and disability will encounter gray areas in definitions and evaluations; terms such as "impairment" and "disability" are used in different settings to mean the same thing and, at other times, to mean two different things, as you can see in Table 7.3. Later in this chapter, we

Table 7.3 Four conceptual components of disability

Pathology	Interruption/interference with bodily process or structure
Impairment	Loss of psychological, anatomical or physiological structure or function
Functional limitation	Inability, from impairment, to perform activity within the normal range
Disability	Inability to perform usual activities from impairment—task specific

will look at individual disability systems in the United States and their basic requirements. But first, let us look at the lexicon of disability shown in Table 7.3.

Pathology

Pathology is a disease or trauma that causes changes in the structure or function of the body. When used in the context of disability, pathology refers to an interruption or interference with a normal bodily process or structure. The term includes the initial injury to the body from trauma, infection, metabolic disorder or other etiology, and the body's response to such injury. *Thus, pathology is at the tissue level.* Pathology also includes aggravation of a previously existing problem by an injury. Examples of pathology include lumbosacral strain, herniated lumbar disk disease, and diabetic polyneuropathy.

Impairment

Impairment is defined as any loss or abnormality of psychological, anatomical, or physiological structure or function. It may be temporary, during active pathology, or may become permanent, continuing even after the pathological process is adequately treated and resolved. *Thus, impairments are at the organ level.*

Examples of impairments include decreased range of motion from lumbosacral strain or herniated lumbar disk, altered reflexes, decreased strength or loss of sensation from radiculopathy or abnormal electromyography studies seen in a person with a herniated disk or diabetic polyneuropathy. Anatomic impairments include contractures, loss of limb/amputation, deformities, and decreased range of motion. Physiologic impairments include decreased cardiac output, decreased pulmonary function, abnormal electrophysiologic studies, abnormal blood chemistry, and muscle weakness.

Impairment also includes changes in cognition and memory, as seen in persons with closed head injury, and abnormalities of personality detected on the Minnesota Multiphasic Personality Inventory 2 (MMPI 2) which offers objective evidence of psychological impairments. It is important to recognize that *impairments are objective and medically determinable through clinical or laboratory assessments.*

Functional Limitation(s)

Functional limitation is a restriction in or lack of ability to perform an activity or function in a manner that is within the range considered normal for that person and that results from impairment. Examples of functional limitations include the inability to lift more than 20 lb by an individual with lumbosacral disk and nerve decompression; the inability to follow a two-step direction in a person with head trauma; the inability to do exertional activities, such as climbing stairs in a person with ischemic heart disease; and the inability to function safely in the community in a person with cognitive or affective changes resulting from a closed head injury. *Thus, functional limitations are manifestations of impairment, translated in terms of the function of a body part or organ.*

Disability

Disability is defined as the inability of a person to perform his or her usual activities and the inability to assume one's usual obligations. It is any restriction or lack (resulting from impairment) of the ability to perform an activity in the manner or within in the range considered normal for a human being. *Disability is task specific.* Permanent disability is assumed to be present if a patient's actual or presumed ability to engage in gainful activity is reduced or absent as a result of an impairment, which in turn may or may not be combined with other factors. *Disability is at the person level.*

   This framework for understanding disability derives from international classifications of impairment, disability and handicap drafted decades ago that include (1) disease, (2) impairment, (3) disability, and (4) handicap (Vasudevan and Ajuwon 2005). Disease is a pathological condition of the body, whereas impairment is the loss of normal anatomic, physiologic, or psychological status. Disability, in this context, is loss of normal function that is task specific and handicap is defined as a loss of normal function that is role specific. Examples of handicap include limited access to public facilities though, increasingly, environmental modifications in work settings and the community can decrease handicap. To summarize, pathology is at the tissue level, impairment is at the organ level, disability at the person level, and handicap at the societal level.

   Clearly, the four concepts also interrelate and affect each other. Aggressive treatment of pathology may eliminate or minimize permanent impairments and aggressive treatment of impairments can decrease functional limitations. Limited function can be enhanced by assistive and adaptive devices and acceptance of limitations, through counseling, can decrease a patient's disability conviction. Multidisciplinary care versus isolated, expensive and uncoordinated care models also encourages greater focus on "abilities" than on "disability."

Functional Capacity Assessments

In disability medicine, there is also significant confusion between evaluative tests known as "work capacity evaluation," "physical capacity evaluation," "functional musculoskeletal evaluation," "ergonomic job analysis," "maximum lifting limits," "functional capacity assessment" (FCA) and "functional capacity evaluation."

Most of these tests measure a patient's residual functional capacity to capably sustain dependable performance in response to a broadly defined work demands. The evaluation should be based on a patient's present medical, physical, and psychological state, not the patient's physical potential. Because of the lack of accepted definitions and procedures for such evaluations to determine disability, many providers offer "FCAs" which have become a profitable growth industry (Genovese and Galper 2011). Clinicians should exercise some caution when ordering and analyzing such tests.

The Disability Evaluation Process

Just as it is difficult to verify pain in a patient, it is difficult to determine disability. This is especially true in patients presenting with only pain as the causative factor in their disability. Yet both conditions respond well to the rehabilitation process and there is ample evidence of the effectiveness of the multidisciplinary pain treatment in decreasing, if not reversing, the disability associated with chronic pain. In treating pain-related disability, the focus should be on improving function with clear goal setting. Notably, *assessment of permanent disability should not occur until the patient has completed adequate and appropriate rehabilitation or if the patient declines appropriate psychosocial and multidisciplinary treatment.*

The basis of disability evaluation frequently depends on the physician's ability to assess "medically determinable and objective impairments." But, assessment of disability is hindered by differing opinions and approaches of physicians. For example, studies have demonstrated that physicians' evaluations of patients with low back pain, especially based on nonneurological findings, such as muscle spasm and guarding, diverge widely (Waddell et al. 1982).

In addition to physical examinations which are not always an objective and consistent method of determining impairment, radiologic abnormalities are not always useful. As we saw in previous chapters, problems revealed on imaging frequently lack clinical correlation with symptoms. Beware the "X-ray diagnosis."

There also exists a poor relationship and lack of correlation between objectively demonstrable pathology and an individual patient's functional level and disability says the Institute of Medicine on the basis of literature reviews (1987).

Assessment of permanent disability should not occur until the patient has completed adequate and appropriate rehabilitation

---

As early as 1979, Grossman noted that subjective differences in clinical evaluations occur because disability as a concept was viewed differently by various professionals who participated in formulating the concept (Grossman 1979). He compared the disability evaluation process to the fable of three blind men asked to describe an elephant, each having touched only one part of the elephant's anatomy, and thus viewing things extremely differently. Grossman also pointed out the irony that a patient's pain symptoms, acknowledged by a treating physician, are at times *not* admissible in court, whereas testimony from physicians *not* treating the patient frequently is allowed.

Finally, patients themselves can present challenges when they have disabilities. Many of the biopsychosocial processes seen with chronic pain are more pronounced in patients with disabilities including fear of pain (anticipatory pain), confusing "hurt" with "harm" when they feel pain, high levels of anger, resentment and stress, and intense family dynamics. Like other chronic pain patients, patients with disabilities tend to have

1. Pain persisting beyond the expected healing period of an injury or illness, excluding cancer
2. Pain with minimal objective clinical and laboratory findings or residual structural effects that can explain the pain behavior
3. Pain that lacks specific and clear medical or surgical interventions to treat the underlying problem
4. Pain associated with sedentary lifestyle changes

But medical professionals can also contribute to the biopsychosocial processes that complicate pain treatment. Bishop et al. (2007) found that when clinicians subscribed to a strong "patho-anatomical" approach, believing in strong links between pain and impairment, biomedical rather than multidisciplinary treatment and that "hurt is harm," patients were much more likely to have the same beliefs and engage in fear avoidance. Linton et al. also found some clinicians stoking patients' fear avoidance through their belief that sick leave was an *actual treatment* for patients, thus reinforcing their disability behaviors (Linton et al. 2002). *Instead, clinicians should recognize that "disability" is a behavioral response which, like pain, can be a "learned behavior"* (see Chaps. 3 and 4), and therefore should encourage patients to stay active and avoid excessive rest, return to work, and learn and practice self-management with their pain (Bishop et al. 2007).

Employers' Role in Disability

Employers are clearly "ground zero" when it comes to disabled workers but they could do more to *prevent* disabling worker events through a shift in perspective from "traditional interventions that treat or rehabilitate the individual, to a more holistic approach to workers' health," says Waddell et al. (2008). While accepting that common health problems are an inevitable part of working life, "good occupational management is about preventing persistent and disabling consequences" and encouraging "an environment that "allows workers to maintain and improve their health and well-being," says Waddell. The philosophical switch is shown in Table 7.4.

Employers, unions, and insurers need to rethink workplace conditions such that there is early detection and treatment of workers' mild to moderate symptoms, accommodation of functional limitations, and recurrent symptoms and interventions to facilitate return to work. Employers also need to develop, implement, and disseminate a clear sickness and absence policy for their workers and management, as shown in Table 7.5.

As we often note in this book, patients should be educated early and often about the difference between the terms "hurt" which implies pain or discomfort and "harm" which implies injury/damage. Too often the terms are used interchangeably by patients, clinicians, and the healthcare industry, and they are philosophically very different.

Table 7.4 Toward a new workplace philosophy

Old thinking	New thinking
Common health problems lead to disability	Common health problems are manageable
Solutions are found in healthcare system	Solutions are held by all stakeholders
Work is inherently risky	Work is good for physical, mental health
Ill workers need protection from work	Work is therapeutic; work prevents feelings of worthlessness

Table 7.5 Desirable features of employer sick/absence plan

Clear corporate policy	Includes recording/monitoring of absences
Senior management commitment	Training/auditing of supervisors, managers
Detection of early problems	Especially when symptoms are mild to moderate
Accommodation	"Job crafting" for functional limitations when possible
Maintain worker contact	Early and continued contact through absence
Connect worker with services	Occupational therapy, psychologists, more
Substitute temporary work	Offer modified work if available
Involve worker in decisions	Especially the planning process for return to work

Once the patient with pain, especially chronic pain, recognizes and accepts that certain activities recommended by the physician or physical therapist may increase pain (hurt), but will not cause damage or reinjury (harm), he begins the important journey from "pain-related disability" to higher levels of activities and function.

Instead of the old adage "If it hurts, don't do it," "If it hurts, rest" and "Use pain as your guide," the hurt-is-not-harm distinction is a new paradigm that supports patients in increasing their activities and decreasing their disability behaviors and enactment of a "disabled role." This process, which encourages patients to move toward less disability behaviors and toward an improved quality of life, is sometimes referred to as a "boot-camp approach" or a "sports medicine approach of graded increase in activity." Appropriate pharmacological agents, including analgesics, should be used to help patients "continue with activities" (Linton et al. 2002).

Needless to say, when there are monetary awards at stake from work-related or traffic-related injuries or accidents, there can be a "secondary gain" for patients to continue their disability behaviors, often inadvertently and rarely consciously. These tendencies can be supported by patients' families.

Lack of job satisfaction and security and lack of support from employers or union shops can also add to the disability conviction and illness and pain "behaviors." All of these myriad of factors affect a patient's recovery and return to work as seen in Table 7.6.

Many patients with disabilities have tried unsuccessful medical and surgical treatments and undergone significant lifestyle changes. They often present with disability that exceeds the underlying, identifiable pathologies and the characteristic "D's" associated with it: disuse, dysfunction, deconditioning, drug misuse, depression, and disability.

In fact, patients with disabilities account for a greater level of medication consumption, hospital admissions, and physician visits than the general population and even greater suicide rates. They have usually received unimodal treatments, such as

Table 7.6 Barriers to returning to work	
	Poor general health
	Poor mental health
	Excessive medication
	Anticipatory fear of pain
	Anger
	Resentment
	Stress
	Family factors
	Monetary gain
	Nonsupport from employer
	Nonsupport from union
	Unimodal care (repeat surgeries, injections, opioids)
	Lack of psychological services

excessive opioids and repeated surgeries and have not been offered the needed and appropriate psychological services which characterize multidisciplinary rehabilitative care.

Some studies, such as those conducted by the Boeing Company, suggest biopsychosocial factors have a greater predictive power for future disability than biomechanical or ergonomic measures in many work settings. Measures of job happiness and personality measures were better predictors of future back pain than physical factors. Those who measured lower on job happiness scales were 2.5 times more likely to file back injury reports and those with higher scores on scale 3 (the so-called "hysteria" scale) of the MMPI were twice as likely to file back injury reports compared with those who had lower scores. Age and gender were not as clear determinants as these psychological factors (Fordyce 1995; Loeser 1980).

The International Association for the Study of Pain's task force on pain in the workplace has found that healthcare providers themselves can play a major role in creating disability and that "fewer than 15 % of persons with back pain can be assigned to one of these categories of specific low back pain" (Fordyce 1995). Noting the many defects in determination of disability, medically and legally which often confound compensation awards, Fordyce suggests use of the term *activity intolerance* instead of disability for cases where pain is the main reason behind dysfunction.

Several years ago, Weinstein observed the sociological transformation that can occur with disability: an unacceptable disability, equated with weakness and failure, is transformed into an acceptable disability which is neither dishonorable nor shameful through the "accident process" (Weinstein 1978). He observed that the first phase of the disability process includes a period of tension and stress, in which the worker experiences an unwelcome dysphoric state that includes frustration, insecurity, and feelings of incompetence. The second phase is often characterized by the worker's experience and sometimes denial of dependency and passivity which the patient is unable to accept and acknowledge.

The third phase of the disability process, says Weinstein, is the *injury* which transforms the worker into someone who is impaired and needs help. Because the injurious effects have occurred as the result of an externally generated event, something that "could happen to anyone," sympathy is afforded to the worker from family, friends, and likely coworkers. Thus, the brief accident process transfers an unacceptable disability into an acceptable one. In the final phase of this process, disability can become a way of life unless multidisciplinary care is offered to the worker/patient. When viewed in this way, a work-related disability is the end result of a *complex process* rather than a direct consequence of a discrete accident or illness.

Systems of Disability

Most medical professionals, especially physicians, who see pain patients will be asked to complete forms for them, their attorneys or insurance carriers at some point in their practice. We are often asked to assess the causation of disability and the prospect of a patient returning to work, so it is important to have a basic familiarity with the different systems. The information in this section is not intended as a substitute for specific information from the state where you practice or programs affecting your patient.

The United States' disability programs and systems include:

1. Workers' Compensation insurance, usually regulated by each state
2. Social Security Disability Insurance and Supplemental Social Security (federal programs)
3. The Veterans Administration, compensation, and pension benefits
4. Private disability insurance

Other disability-related programs also exist, associated with the Federal Employers Liability Act, the Jones Act (Merchant Marine), the Longshore and Harbor Workers' Compensation Act, the Federal Black Lung Benefits Program, the American with Disabilities Act, the Federal Employees' Compensation Act, the FMLA, the Department of Veterans Affairs/Vocational Rehabilitation Assistance, the Department of Workforce Development Disability and private disability and tort/personal injury law.

While the requirements of the programs obviously differ, medical professionals are usually relied upon to determine:

1. Causation of the injury and the relationship of the injury to pathology/disease
2. Identification of appropriate anatomic, physiologic, and psychological impairments after Maximum Medical Improvements (MMI) also called end of healing or "healing plateau" in Workers' Compensation systems.
3. Identification of the functional limitations imposed by the *permanent* impairments
4. Relationship of functional limitations to the individual's work activities (and other personal activities in personal injury case) and future work responsibilities (in work-related injuries) as well as other recreational and social activities in other settings.
5. Suggestions for future treatment and rehabilitation
6. Permanency of impairment (or disability rating in most Workers' Compensation systems) and statements — whether the impairments are expected to last up to 12 months or to be permanent (specifically in determination of Social Security benefits).
7. The percentage of disability compared with the "whole person" or to the "scheduled part of the body" in Workers' Compensation system.

At a minimum, most disability reports will also include:

1. History of injuries and illnesses
2. History of treatment for the presenting problem
3. Medical, family, educational, work, and social history
4. A description of the patient's present pain status and its effect on physical, psychological, social, economic and vocational status

5. A detailed neuromusculoskeletal examination (depending on the system involved)
6. Medical diagnosis
7. Summary of objective findings supporting diagnosis
8. Description of impairments
9. Description of functional limitations imposed by the impairments
10. Relationship between functional limitations and work activities
11. Relationship between functional limitations and activities of daily living, social, and recreational activities
12. Causal relationship between injury and impairments
13. Determination of duration of impairments (permanent)—after appropriate medical, surgical, physical, and psychological approaches have been exhausted and a "healing plateau" and MMI have been reached
14. Recommendations for future treatment, including medications, equipment, environmental modification, medical and surgical needs and rehabilitation needs
15. Expected future course of the condition and its prognosis, especially regarding stability
16. Percentage of impairment and disability, depending on the system involved

Clearly, you will need to understand the difference between "disability" and "impairment" and the definitions of other related terms to provide this information. While the opinions of other medical professionals may be sought, once a patient has reached "Maximum Medical Treatment" (MMI) or a "healing plateau," the point where no additional benefit is expected from further treatment, the treating physician is usually the best suited to evaluate the patient's disability.

Some disability systems and jurisdictions seek a confirmation of "reasonable degree of medical certainty" from medical professionals. Although this may be formidable for physicians because we are never "certain" of any diagnosis, it is important to understand that, from a medicolegal perspective, "certainty" can be seen to refer to "probability." A "reasonable degree of medical probability," means "more than 51 % likely" which most of us are comfortable asserting.

Medical professionals' "certainty" parallels that of other legal players in the courtroom says (ButieRitchie 2005). "One obvious example [is] juries are not required to be absolutely certain about the guilt of a defendant in a criminal trial."

Tort Claims/Personal Injury System

The United States inherited most of its common law from England where civil cases were decided based on precedent/prior decisions and depended on the legal doctrine of *stari decisis*, which means "let the decision stand" (Vasudevan and Ajuwon 2014). Of the different disability systems, common law is most applicable to the civil tort system. A tort is defined as a "breach of duty that gives rise to an action for damages" and civil wrongdoing. There are four elements of a claim that must be proved before an adjudicating authority and establish (1) a legal duty existed, (2) breach of legal duty occurred, (3) the breach of duty was the proximate or direct cause of harm or injury and (4) harm or damage occurred as a result. Table 7.7 shows examples of tort cases and Table 7.8, the types of determinations that can be made in this system.

Tort cases usually arise out of

1. Personal injury caused by motor vehicle accidents
2. Product liability due to defective products
3. Medical negligence/malpractice
4. Toxic exposure
5. Slip and fall cases

In the United States, the Seventh Amendment of the Constitution upholds tort law, ruling that, "In suits at common law, where the value in controversy shall exceed twenty Dollars, the right of trial by jury shall be preserved." Of course, no controversy today would be *less* than twenty dollars.

In the tort system, the physician is pivotal in providing information about the diagnosis, its causal relationship with the injury, the required treatment, future care, permanent impairments, if any, and their effect on a patient's vocational and other activities. If you are not used to this system, it can be intimidating. You will find yourself participating in discovery, trial depositions and sometimes even required to

Table 7.7 Examples of tort cases

Personal injury due to motor vehicle accidents
Product liability due to defective products
Medical negligence/malpractice
Toxic exposure
Slip and fall cases

Table 7.8 Determinations within the tort system

Liability	Who was at fault for injury/disease (the medical profession does not determine this)
Causality	Did preexisting or underlying conditions exist? Was the preexisting condition aggravated, accelerated or precipitated by injury? Was injury direct and proximate to the diagnosis?
Relationship	What findings are directly related to the injury?
Improvement	Has patient reached maximum improvement; end of healing?
Residual Impairments	What objective impairments persist despite optimal treatment?
Functional Limitations	What are patient's task-specific disabilities?
Prognosis	What care will patient need in future?

be present in court with a judge or a jury trial if mediation and out-of-court settle-ment fail to settle the case.

Findings of medical negligence frequently center around the four concepts of (1) duty, (2) dereliction, (3) direct cause, and (4) damages.

Duty exists when the physician–patient relationship has been established. The patient has sought the assistance of the physician and the physician knowingly has undertaken to provide the needed medical service.

Dereliction, the second element required in medical negligence, implies failure to perform duty. There must be proof that the physician neglected the duty to the patient and that there was deviation from a standard of care.

Direct Cause requires that there be proof that the harm to the patient was directly caused by the physician, his actions or failure to act and that the harm would not otherwise have occurred.

Damages and losses that the patient sustained from actions of the physician must be established.

Frequently, physician-prepared Independent Medical Examinations (IME) (or Adversarial Medical Examinations as they are sometimes called), play a key part in tort proceedings. While some physicians restrict themselves to either working with the plaintiff or the defense side, others may attempt to develop a "middle of the road" reputation and to work with both sides. Still, a medical professional can be "branded" as a plaintiff or defense expert, irrespective of the care they take in being consistent and objective.

It is therefore very important to be "consistent" and "independent" in your exam-ination and reports, irrespective of the party requesting your medical opinion. If additional, new or contrary medical information is provided, you should be willing to change your opinions and willing to present your medical rationale for changing or not changing your opinions. I have personally testified in trials in which material unknown to me was presented that nullified or altered my original opinion and I have not been afraid to humbly change my opinion on the basis of the new evidence. If you find yourself involved in legal proceedings, try to remember that juries are welcoming and accepting of such humility. A jury is likely to be much less sympathetic to a physician who sticks to an opinion that is now in doubt and refuses to be humble.

A physician working within the tort system will often be asked to make the following determinations. (Note: Physicians and medical professionals have no role in the legal determination of *liability* in most personal injury cases, such as from a "slip and fall" or motor vehicle accident incident; that is, who or what was the cause of an injury/disease.)

Causality

Did the accident/event cause a medical diagnostic condition or was there an under-lying or preexisting condition that was substantially aggravated? In the questions of causation and subsequent issues, the physician/medical professional has a very important role. This can be a very difficult and controversial opinion (see references; "Determination of causation.")

Relationship

Which of the medical evaluations and treatment that followed the accident or event are directly related to the injury?

Improvement

Has the patient reached MMI or a healing plateau, where additional treatment or time is not expected to result in significant additional improvement?

Residual Impairments

What are the residual impairments (objectively determined medical findings) resulting from the injury/event and are they permanent? Pain by itself is a symptom and is not an objective impairment.

Functional Limitations

How do the impairments contribute to alteration of functional activities, both in work and in social/recreational activities? In other words what are the patient's task-specific abilities/disabilities? Do the functions that are restricted, result in safety issues for the individual with injury or coworkers?

Prognosis

Is there need for ongoing treatment for the patient and is it directly related to the injury or event? If so what specific treatment? Is the condition stable?

Workers' Compensation System

The Workers' Compensation system is the most common litigation system for a physician treating patients with pain arising from work-related injuries, and, in the United States it dates back to 1911. Before that time, the only way that an injured worker could obtain compensation after an injury at work was through the just-reviewed tort system. The injured worker, or plaintiff, was and is usually at a disadvantage in the tort system because of the time and expense required and powerful strategies used by the employers and insurers. These defense strategies include:

1. **Contributory Negligence**
   Defendants seek to show an employee was himself at fault
2. **Assumption of Risk**
   Defendants seek to show that an injury was related to the inherent risk or hazard of the job of which the worker knew or *should have known*
3. **The "Fellow Servant" Doctrine**
   Defendants seek to prove that the injury occurred due to negligent actions of *fellow workers* and not management.

With these defense strategies, it has been difficult, if not impossible, for injured workers to obtain adequate compensation for work-related injuries, a situation which provided impetus and rationale for the development of today's Workers' Compensation system in the United States originally called the Workman's Compensation Act, Wisconsin was the first state to enact the legislation followed by New York and New Jersey. By 1949, all states had enacted a Workers' Compensation law, which is mandatory in almost all states. Rondinelli and Katz and other researchers whose publications are found at the end of this chapter under references have traced the origins and development of Workers' Compensation laws in the United States. The main disability classifications in the Workers' Compensation system are shown in Table 7.9.

The Workers' Compensation program is based on a "no fault" system which provides automatic coverage to employees who make a claim for "injuries that arises out of and in the course of employment," in exchange for employees waiving their right to sue the employer. Exceptions for the waiver exist, however, for "wanton neglect" by employers and third party lawsuits (Vasudevan and Ajuwon 2005).

Not everyone is a fan of the US Workers' Compensation system. Nortin Hadler, M.D., author of *Stabbed in the Back: Confronting Back Pain in an Overtreated Society* (2009) calls it a "scheme" that medicalizes non-injuries. "The notion of a 'ruptured disk' found footing in Workers' Compensation, but rapidly became part of the common sense. People could have a backache and exclaim 'I injured my back.' Furthermore, the labeling as a ruptured disk ushered in the surgical era of disk

Table 7.9 Major categories in US Workers' Compensation

TTD	Temporary Total Disability
TPD	Temporary Partial Disability
PPD	Permanent Partial Disability
PTD	Permanent Total Disability
Scheduled PPD	Affects limbs, eyes and ears
Unscheduled PPD	Affects spine, head, and torso

surgery and the common sense that people have 'bad backs' and suffer 'wear and tear,' he writes. In fact, says Dr. Hadler, the so-called injuries are not injuries all but "regional backache" that do not denote neurological damage and the patients are "otherwise well."

There are several benefits found within the Workers' Compensation system including survivor benefits in cases of death, medical and rehabilitation expenses, wage loss benefits and monetary compensation. Most state programs provide medical and rehabilitation treatment to "cure and relieve" the effects of a worker's injury. Wage loss compensation benefits in the US Workers' Compensation system are based on the category of disability. While an employee is under active treatment, the categories can include Temporary Total Disability (TTD) and Temporary Partial Disability (TPD). Once a worker reaches End of Healing, also called a healing plateau, or MMI, he is eligible for benefits for residual Permanent Partial Disability (PPD) or Permanent Total Disability (PTD). A PPD designation can be "Scheduled," denoting injuries to limbs, eyes, ears, or "Unscheduled" denoting injuries to the spine, head, and torso. The input of medical professionals in deciding these categories is crucial.

Similar to what is found in the tort system, in the Workers' Compensation, physicians are called upon to evaluate a worker's medical condition and to what extent it was affected by events or accidents in the workplace. *Key concepts in this determination are "medical probability"—that an injury was more likely than not (51% or greater) caused by a certain event as opposed to "medical possibility" in which an injury was unlikely (less than 50%) caused by a certain event*, shown in Table 7.10. (Remember, Workers' Compensation is a "no fault" system so liability is not an issue.)

In addition to determining causality, physicians in the Workers' Compensation system provide their opinion about where in the disability process their patient is, treatment(s) the injury/event required and when a patient has reached MMI as shown in Table 7.10.

Most Workers' Compensation injuries are appropriately diagnosed and treated and conclude with full "Resolution" or "Minimal Impairment" ratings and appropriate compensation, as needed. However, it must be noted that 10–20 % of Workers' Compensation injuries contribute to over *80% of the costs* in the program and contributing to this is the contentious, adversarial process that is sometimes involved. One clear reason is that physicians frequently arrive at very conflicting opinions based

Table 7.10 Determinations with the Workers' Compensation system	
Causality
Stage of disability
Required treatment(s)
Maximum Medical Improvement or end of healing
Future medical treatment
Date of end of healing
Permanent restrictions, if any
Percentage of disability scheduled or unscheduled (body as a whole)

on their own background and philosophies. In these cases, Independent Medical Evaluations are valuable legal remedies available to the insurance companies and a "second opinion" is available to the injured worker.

Private Disability Programs

Many but not all employers provide short-term and long-term disability for their employees. If you are asked to fill out a form when you see a patient, it is often for these employers.

Short-Term Disability

After an illness like influenza or pneumonia or an asthma flare up, elective or emergency surgery or injuries such as fractures, strains/sprains, an employee is often unable to work on a short-term basis. In these situations, you may be asked to write a note on your medical practice's letterhead indicating the patient's medical condition and that he was "disabled from work" during the time period in question— allowing him to be eligible for short-term disability (STD) benefits. Although contractual language can vary, many employers provide employees up to 90 days in short-term disability, which is usually enough time for minor injuries and illnesses to resolve.

Long-Term Disability

When the period of disability exceeds a few months and a health condition or event is not covered by Workers' Compensation, some employers offer long-term disability programs that typically cover an employee for a year (12 months) from the initial date of disability. The forms to activate these programs may be sent to you or the patient may bring them to the office to be filled out and mailed to the respective party. The information you may be required to provide is shown in Table 7.7.

These forms typically pose simple questions such as the name and date of birth of the patient and cause/diagnosis of the patient's disability from work, the date the disability started, surgery or hospitalization dates, if applicable and the names of other medical professions treating the patient. Sometimes long-term disability forms ask when a patient will recover and/or return to full duty work without restrictions, what kind of work he can perform and what his prognosis is—questions that can be frustrating because of the many "unknowns" and ambiguities in disability and pain medicine. However, instead of skipping such questions, it is best to answer

Table 7.11 Information
needed in private disability
systems

Medical diagnosis
Dates of disability from a certain date to a certain date
Date when treatment began
Dates when patient was totally disabled
Expected date of return to restricted work
Expected date of return to unrestricted work
Expected length of total or temporary disability
Accommodations to facilitate return to work, if any

"I do not know" or a nuanced answer like, "this is difficult to determine at this time but I anticipate recovery and return to previous work in two months."

It is important that you fill out your patient's forms, whether from an employer, third parties or pertaining to auto insurance or school loans, in a timely fashion to not delay your patient's disability payments. The forms are time consuming but they are part of the thorough medical care we are sworn to provide and our role as a patient advocate.

Once a patient is on long-term disability, in many private disability plans the criteria of reemployment may change from return to "previous work" to the "ability for any occupation." In some situations, the private disability criteria for assistance after expiration of LTD benefits, is similar to Social Security and programs which we will explore shortly. A few individual, private disability policies are available that will provide greater duration of protection and disability payments for higher premiums if an individual cannot resume performance of his previous job over an extended period of time or indefinitely due to a medically determined diagnostic condition. Information commonly required in private disability systems is shown in Table 7.11.

Family Medical Leave Act

The FMLA was enacted in 1993 to provide up to 12 weeks of unpaid leave due to "medical necessity." While often associated with the birth or adoption of a child, the act may apply to either gender. Administered by the Wage and Hour Division of the United States Department of Labor, the act also provides unpaid leave for the care of immediate family members or an employee's own illness.

The FMLA forms can be long and confusing, but when appropriately filled and signed by a physician, they allow the patient to take unpaid time off work without having to use sick days. The forms allow medical professionals to designate treatment that has been provided for a medical condition or flare up of a medical condition over a period of several months including physical therapy, injections, or counseling.

The Social Security Systems

The Social Security Administration (SSA) is the largest disability program in the United States, assisting up to half of all persons qualified as disabled (Vasudevan and Ajuwon 2005). Included in the SSA is the Social Security Disability Insurance (SSDI), a program established in 1956 to create a fund for workers who were permanently disabled, funded through payroll taxes. Generally, applicants for SSDI begin at the state level with the Bureau of Disability Determination. To be eligible they must have worked in a job covered by SSDI for a minimum period preceding the onset of disability. Pension benefits are available to those determined to be totally disabled.

Another SSA disability program is the Supplemental Social Security Income (SSI) system. SSI provides benefits to disabled individuals whose income and assets meet minimum criteria according to a "means test." Unlike, SSDI, SSI is funded through general revenue and does not require that the applicant have a certain work history for eligibility.

Both SSDI and SSI are based on "medically determinable impairments," which are defined as "An impairment that results from anatomical, physiological or psychological abnormalities which can be shown by medically acceptable clinical and laboratory diagnostic techniques." A physical or mental impairment must be established with laboratory findings and other medical evidence in addition to signs and symptomatology.

Social Security Disability Insurance

The SSDI system is an "All or None" disability system. The disability determination is decided by a disability examiner through the Local Disability Determination office and a hearing examiner. Monthly income support benefits are available for people under age 65 who meet certain working criteria in the last 20 out of last 40 quarters which include:

1. Their medical condition is severely incapacitating so that they are unable to "Engage in any Substantial Gainful Activity" (SGA) because of medically determinable physical or mental impairment that can be expected to "result in death" or that has lasted or can be expected to last for a continuous period of not more than 12 months.
2. They are widows or widowers of a covered individual who meets the definition of disability
3. They are disabled offspring (children or adult) of a covered individual who meets the definition of disability

After an applicant for SSDI has completed all forms and forwarded all pertinent medical information to his treating physicians, a medical consultant from the SSA will examine the claimant and provide further medical information that will be used in the disability determination process. "Residual Functional Capacities" forms are included in the determinations.

The application has a sequential five-step process in which the medical opinions of the treating physicians and especially medically based objective evidence of impairments play a significant role. Unlike most Workers' Compensation or personal injury cases, a physician's notes that a patient is disabled, *unless supported by objective documentation*, are of no value. It is especially challenging, therefore, for physicians to supply SSA with acceptable documentation of lumbar conditions, fibromyalgia and common but vague pain conditions like complex regional pain syndrome.

Supplemental Security Income

The Supplemental Security Income (SSI) program applies the same medical criteria as SSDI but, unlike SSDI, does not require prior work history for eligibility. Cash transfers under SSI are substantially smaller than under SSDI and are contingent on the beneficiary having very low income and assets. Medical coverage under SSI is provided through Medicaid rather than Medicare (which accompanies SSDI) and recipients of SSI seldom return to work.

The Medical Professional's Role in Disability

The role of the medical professional will differ depending upon which disability system is involved. For example, the physician's role in SSA programs is much more limited than that found in Workers' Compensation, personal injury and tort systems. Primary care physicians are frequently asked by their patients to help them "get Social Security benefit" only to find their notes and findings determining that the person is disabled hold no sway and are of no value without other documentation.

In legal situations, it is important to remember that you are a medical professional not a lawyer. When you are preparing for conferences with attorneys, depositions, interrogatories or speaking with experts about liability, causation and damages, it is important to listen to and cooperate with defense attorney and insurance staff but never discuss the case with others. Needless to say, you should *never alter medical records*.

With all disability systems, the patient comes first whether we are helping with compensation, return to work or both (though we never falsely attribute an injury to work). As with all chronic pain patients, you should encourage the patient to continue his ordinary activities, stay active, and maintain his recovery goals. It is important to ask the patient about his job, duties, and plans for returning to work and to make psychological help available.

Table 7.12 Main points of this chapter

Unimodal treatment of disabilities delays return to work
As with chronic pain, biopsychosocial factors are key in disability
Learn terminology like the difference between disability and impairment
Factual and legal challenges complicate disability evaluation
Workers' Compensation, Social Security are leading disability systems
Put patient needs first especially return to work and functionality

References

Bishop, A., Foster, N., Thomas, E., & Hay, E. (2007). How does the self-reported clinical management of patients with low back pain relate to the attitudes and beliefs of health care practitioners? *Pain, 135*, 187–195.

Burns, J., Sherman, M. L., Devine, J., Mahoney, N., & Pawl, R. (2005). Association between Workers' compensation and outcome following multidisciplinary treatment for chronic pain. *The Clinical Journal of Pain, 11*, 94–102.

ButieRitchie, D. T. (2005). "Objectively speaking…" there is no such thing in the law! *Disability Medicine, 5*(1), 6–12.

Dworkin, R. H., Handlin, D. S., Richlin, D. M., Brand, L., & Vannucci, C. (1985). Unraveling the effects of compensation, litigation, and employment on treatment response in chronic pain. *Pain, 23*(1), 49–59.

Fauber, J. (2012, October 2). Many injured workers remain on opioids, study finds. *Journal Sentinel.*

Fordyce, W. (Ed.). (1995). Back pain in the work place: Management of disability in nonspecific 723 conditions. Report of the task force on pain in the work place. Seattle, WA: International 724 Association for the Study of Pain.

Genovese, E., & Galper, J. S. (2011). In R. Gatchel (Ed.), *Guide to the evaluation of functional ability.* New York: Springer.

Grossman, H. I. (1979). A new concept of disability. *Journal of Rehabilitation, 45*, 41–49.

Hadler, N. (2008). *Worried sick* (1st ed., p. 118). Charlotte: The University of North Carolina Press.

International Association for the Study of Pain. (1995). *Back pain in the work place: Management of disability in nonspecific conditions.* Report of the task force on pain in the work place, Seattle, WA.

Jacks, P. (1994 June). Malingering & fraud in psychiatric Workers' Compensation claims. *California Workers' Compensation Enquirer.*

Linton, S., Viaeyen, J., & Ostelo, R. (2002). The back pain beliefs of health care providers. *Journal of Occupational Rehabilitation, 12*(4), 223–232.

Loeser, G. D. (1980). In J. P. Turner (Ed.), *Perspectives on pain in Proceedings of the First World Congress on Clinical Pharmacology and Therapeutic* (pp. 315–326). London: MacMillan.

Meier, B. (2013, June 23). Profiting from pain. *New York Times.*

National Institute of Neurological Disorders and Stroke. (2014). Low back pain fact sheet.

Nguyen, T., Randolph, D., Talmage, J., Succop, P., & Travis, R. (2010). Long-term outcomes of lumbar fusion among Workers' Compensation subjects. *Spine, 36*(4), 320–321.

Osterweis, M. (1987). *Pain and disability—Clinical, behavioral, and public policy perspective.* Committee on pain, disability and chronic illness behavior. Washington, DC: National Academy Press.

Ranavaya, M. (2012). Primary care physician and prescription narcotics for the treatment of chronic non-malignant pain. *Disability Medicine, 8*(1), 4–6.

Rogers, J., Stout, C., Mack, B., Whitney, N., & Loughran, L. (2013). Return-to-work outcomes in non-operative lumbar cases following an evidence-based post-surgical rehabilitation program. *Disability Medicine, 9*(1), 3–9.

Tait, R. (2013). Presenteeism and pain: Psychosocial and demographic correlates of employment and disability. *Pain Medicine, 14*(11), 1617–1618.

University of North Carolina Press. (2009). Author Q and A. *Stabbed in the back, confronting back pain in an overtreated society.* Retrieved from http://www.uncpress.unc.edu/browse/page/601

Vasudevan, S., & Ajuwon, A. (2014). Disability assessment. In K. Burchiel (Ed.), *Surgical management of pain.* New York: Thieme.

Waddell, G., Burton, A. K., Aylward, M. (2008, May/June). A biopsychosocial model of sickness and disability. *The Guides Newsletter.* American Medical Association.

Waddell, G., Main, C. J., et al. (1982). Normality and reliability in clinical assessment of backache. *British Medical Journal, 284*, 1519–1523.

Weinstein, M. R. (1978). The concept of the disability process. *Psychosomatics, 19*, 94–97.

Further Reading

Genovese, E., & Galper, J. S. (2009). *Guide to the evaluation of functional ability.* Chicago: American Medical Association.

Melhorn, J. M., & Ackerman, W. E. (2009). *Guides to the evaluation of disease and injury causation.* Chicago: American Medical Association.

Melvin, J. L., & Nagi, S. Z. (1970). Factors in behavioral response to impairments. *Archives of Physical Medicine and Rehabilitation., 51*(9), 552–557.

Osterweis, M. (Ed). (1987). *Pain and disability. clinical, behavioral, and public policy perspective.* Committee on pain, disability and chronic illness behavior. Washington, DC: National Academy Press.

Rondinelli, R. D., Genovese, E., & Katz, R. T. (2008). *Guides to the evaluation of permanent impairment* (6th ed.). Chicago: American Medical Association.

Rondinelli, R. D., & Katz, R. T. (2000). *Impairment rating and disability evaluation.* Philadelphia: WB Saunders.

Talmage, J. D. (2007). Failure to communicate: How terminology and phones confuse the work ability/disability evaluation process. *Journal of Insurance Medicine, 39*, 192–198.

Talmage, J. D., & Melhorn, J. M. (2005). *The physician guide to return to work.* Chicago: American Medical Association.

Talmage, J. D., Melhorn, J. M., & Hyman, M. H. (2011). *AMA guides to the evaluation of work ability and return to work.* Chicago: American Medical Association.

Chapter 8
Creating a Multidisciplinary Team

Medical professionals who completed their training since the 1990s, may not remember the golden age of multidisciplinary pain rehabilitation or realize just what a radical concept it was when first developed by John J. Bonica, M.D. Trained as an anesthesiologist, Dr. Bonica noted in a paper written in 1990 that the "specificity theory" (also known as the Door Bell theory, which we review in Chap. 3) resulted in the chemical and surgical interruption of pain pathways, and was the accepted treatment at the early part of the twentieth century. Yet, while working at Madigan Army Hospital in Tacoma, Washington during WWII, he found that "in applying nerve blocks, I noted that while some patients with causalgia [a complex regional pain disorder reviewed in Chap. 10] and other straight-forward pain problems responded to therapy, patients with complex pain problems did not" (Bonica 1990).

Moreover, wrote Dr. Bonica, despite "my efforts to consult textbooks on medicine, neurology, neurosurgery, orthopedics, and other disciplines" he "continued to experience great frustration" in trying to manage complex pain patients "by myself." Even if a patient was seen by different specialists such as an orthopedist, neurologist, and psychiatrist, "it soon became apparent to me that these types of consultation in the isolation of each consultant's office were very slow and inefficient." *The concept of the multidisciplinary approach to pain was thus born.*

Based on positive patient experiences in the 1950s, Dr. Bonica set up a comprehensive multidisciplinary program to treat patients with chronic pain at the University of Washington and Tacoma General Hospital in Seattle, WA. By 1960, the pilot program had evolved into a group of 20 medical professionals from 14 different medical specialties and other healthcare professions. During the same period of time, Benjamin Crue, M.D., founded a similar program in the City of Hope Medical Center in Duarte, CA and a similar program existed in Portland, Oregon founded by William K. Livingston, M.D.

The concept of a multidisciplinary facility for the diagnosis and therapy of complex pain problems was embraced by medical professionals who participated.

© Springer International Publishing Switzerland 2015
S. Vasudevan, *Multidisciplinary Management of Chronic Pain*,
DOI 10.1007/978-3-319-20322-5_8

"Despite numerous problems inherent in individual private practice, for 14 years the group was successful in its objectives and goals," wrote Dr. Bonica. Yet, this new and superior approach for treating pain patients did not catch on right away. "Despite my persistent drum beating, consisting of several hundred lectures and the publication of numerous articles in various parts of the world, the multidisciplinary concept was ignored by the medical profession for two decades," wrote Dr. Bonica. Still, when the medical professional did acknowledge the new pain treatment concept, multidisciplinary pain programs proliferated across the country—so rapidly that they were referred to as "Medicine's new growth industry" (Leff 1976).

John Loeser, M.D., whose Loeser Model of Pain is reviewed in Chap. 3 defines multidisciplinary rehabilitation as including "physical therapy, medication management, education about how the body functions, psychological treatments and learning coping skills, vocational assessment and therapies aimed at improving the likelihood of return to work."

He notes that "the development of multidisciplinary pain programs has been characterized by the shift from the dominant biomedical model of disease to a biopsychosocial model of illness" (Loeser 2014) While multidisciplinary rehabilitation can fail like other chronic pain treatments observes Dr. Loeser, it does not carry the "significant complications" or surgery or "add to the patient's symptoms and signs" when it does not work. Additionally, chronic pain patients "are highly likely to acquire affective and environmental factors that contribute to their complaint of pain," writes Dr. Loeser, "and these are usually not amenable to surgical therapy."

Figure 8.1 shows how multidisciplinary treatment forms the basis of Dr. Loeser's model of pain.

I am proud to say I was part of the golden age of multidisciplinary pain rehabilitation. I inaugurated one of the first multidisciplinary pain programs in the Department of Physical Medicine and Rehabilitation at the Medical College of Wisconsin in 1997, as an outpatient program. By 1984, a fully comprehensive inpatient/outpatient day treatment program and individualized pain center was operating at Elmbrook Memorial Hospital, in Brookfield, Wisconsin, with which I was involved with until 2000. I also had the opportunity to be involved with the Center for Pain and Work Rehabilitation at St. Nicholas Hospital in Sheboygan, Wisconsin from 1990 to through 2013. Over these years, the saying "team work makes the dream work" was proven again and again.

Team Work Makes the Dream Work

Rehabilitation is a team process where multiple individuals from different disciplines help patients achieve their dream.

From 1994 until the writing of this book, I have served as medical director of the Center for Pain Rehabilitation at Community Memorial Hospital in Menomonee Falls, Wisconsin. Our multidisciplinary pain program, based on the principles espoused by Dr. Bonica and his colleagues, still continues in a community clinic of

The Loeser Model of Pain Adapted for Treatment

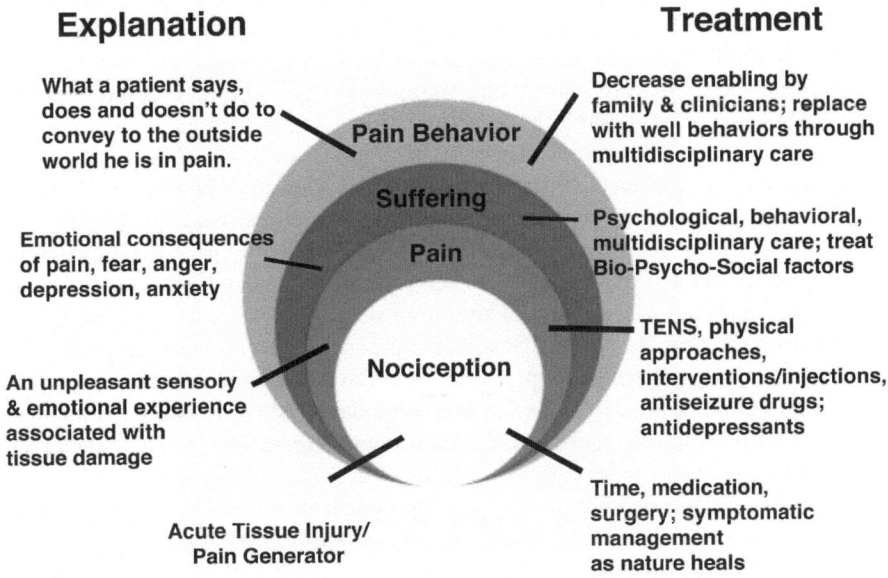

Fig. 8.1 The Loeser model of pain adapted for treatment

the Medical College of Wisconsin in Menomonee Falls, WI, as of the writing of this book. But sadly, as uncoordinated and unimodal pain treatments have supplanted multidisciplinary pain programs, it is one of the few such programs left in the state of Wisconsin.

The Demise of Multidisciplinary Pain Programs

As we have explored in Chaps. 1, 2 and 5, the multidisciplinary pain program pendulum has swung back to the days before Dr. Bonica. The reason is clear—changed reimbursement patterns with increasing emphasis in the healthcare system on unco-ordinated and unimodal care. When discussing nonoperative or conservative care with a colleague, Dr. David Hanscom, author of *Back in Control* recalls that the physician had no exposure at all to multidisciplinary approaches in his medical training (Hanscom 2012). All he had been taught was to "write 'physical therapy' on a prescription pad and send the patient on his or her way," writes Dr. Hanscon. Too many medical professionals graduating today do not even know the definition of conservative (nonoperative) care, writes Dr. Hanscom, *which is 6–12 months of physical therapy visits, 1–3 cortisone injections and "an evaluation by a psychologist who specializes in pain."* Even so, they can be quick to say conservative treatment has "failed" and the next step is surgery without a full grasp of a multidisciplinary approach.

Clearly, "pain clinics" that do not offer a multidisciplinary approach but rather "shot jocks" promoting injections, nerve burnings and excessive surgery have supplanted comprehensive pain programs such as Dr. Bonica and his colleagues originally envisioned. "Pill mills" promoting opioids also have done their part to supplant multidisciplinary care, though the government has begun to regulate such operations and the overuse of opioids in society in general, due to the shocking numbers of opioid abuse-related deaths in the United States, viewed as an epidemic. As we noted in Chap. 5, opioids have no place in the long-term treatment for chronic pain, frequently making pain worse through opioid-induced hyperalgesia" or OIA (Rosenquist 2014). I have personally treated patients who were terrified to titrate off opioids because they were afraid of returning pain, only to find they were in *less pain* once off the opioids. After a decade of unprecedented opioid prescription in the United States, two government-sponsored research papers published in the *Annals of Internal Medicine* in 2015 revealed that there have been only short-term studies of opioid pain relief and there are almost no data supporting their use beyond 6 weeks not to mention the long-term use (Fauber 2015).

The swing of the pendulum is especially concerning because it hails back to older theories of pain which have been cast in doubt by newer ones we know and discuss in Chap. 3. Specifically, cutting and interrupting peripheral body parts to "cover up" pain relies upon the Door Bell theory and ignores more recent and plausible theories including the Matrix Theory of pain, the Spinal Cord Mechanisms theory, the Brain-Based Pain Modulation theory, Neuroimmune Interactions and Pain Genetics. An overview of the major theories of pain is found in Chap. 3. Treatments like blocking the nerve pathway with epidurals, burning nerves to facet joints and surgery to treat normal, age-related degenerative changes of the spine without nerve compression or instability are based on a single, outdated theory of pain. These treatments disregard other significant advances that have occurred in understanding the complex human experience of pain. *When medical professionals ignore the many other theories of pain, it is like they still believe the sun revolves around the earth, a belief popular before Galileo and before the solar system and its complexity were discovered.*

Of all approaches to treating chronic pain, multidisciplinary treatment has the "strongest evidence-base for efficacy, cost-effectiveness, and lack of iatrogenic complications," says the International Society for the Study of Pain (ISAP 2012). This opinion is echoed among other medical associations as well as many government-related groups. Yet, the number of multidisciplinary pain programs has plummeted from 1000 in 1999 to just 150 in 2012 says the ISAP which means there is now only one program per 670,000 in the United States. This is in sharp contrast to 11 European countries and Canada where the number of multidisciplinary pain programs is *increasing*, says ISAP stake holders.

The reason, of course, is obvious. The US healthcare system is financially-driven and "composed of myriad stakeholders says ISAP," notably the insurance industry. In addition to a "pill mentality" which drives the US' huge opioids use, the fact that the US system is for-profit "also speaks to the overutilization of interventional techniques and spinal surgery." Except for the Department of Veterans Affairs, the US health system functions according to the "business ethic" of profitability charges ISAP and has "less concern for human suffering." Yet, adds ISAP, multidisciplinary programs "could potentially save countless billions of dollars every year."

Noting that multidisciplinary programs are not "cash cows" to the institutions that run them, Schatman observed that, "Sadly, while chronic pain management practitioners function under ethical codes of conduct which emphasize the primacy of the patients' well-being, the business ethos and ethics of the healthcare insurance, and hospital corporations may not be directly compatible or supportive of such ethically sound medical care" (Schatman 2006).

We are increasingly seeing a "commodification" of healthcare services in which "surplus provision" is not funded, writes Schatman and multidisciplinary programs find themselves competing with "quick fixes" like opioids for third-party funding. Yet, as we reviewed in Chap. 5, Treatments That Have Questionable or Controversial Evidence, surgery, opioids and blocks, in most cases do not outperform the long-term outcomes of conservative and multidisciplinary care and sometimes are substantially inferior, even as they cost more! "The pharmaceutical approach, alone is often insufficient to treat the multiple and compound issues that instigate and perpetuate a particular patient's pain," Schatman says. Many researchers charge that the United States suffers from "short-termism" in many of its sectors like Wall Street and environmental policy—refusal to look at the long-term costs of immediate actions that appear sensible or profitable. Certainly treating chronic pain with uncoordinated, unimodal care which is not cost-effective when viewed on a long-term basis is another example of such short-term thinking.

There is another irony in the healthcare system embracing chronic pain treatments that are not evidence-based. "Multidisciplinary chronic pain programs place a heavy emphasis on restoring independence to their patients" writes Schatman—yet in the current system, patients lack "the autonomy to choose the treatment which is most likely to restore his or her independence."

Multidisciplinary Pain Programs Have a Strong Evidence-Base

It is not a mystery why multidisciplinary pain programs are effective over the long-term in helping patients manage and control their pain. As we saw in Chap. 3, almost all the pain theories from the Gate Theory to the Matrix, Neuroimmune and Mixmatch theories recognize pain as much more complicated than the simplistic Door Bell Theory (which says when a patient has pain there is a pain generator at

Table 8.1 Multidisciplinary team's treatment goals

Empower patients and family	Education, participation in treatment decisions
Improve function and ADLs	Through knowledge, skills, and training
Reduce dependency on drugs	Eliminate opioids and benzodiazepines; use antidepressant and antiseizure drugs
Reduce dependency on healthcare system	Teach self-management and efficacy
Reduce dependency on family and others	Encourage family and friends to "empathize not sympathize"--not reinforcing pain behaviors
Reduce "pain behaviors"	Replace with "well behaviors"
Return to gainful employment	When possible or even a different job
Improve the quality of life	Including positive attitude, socialization; volunteering; and Reframing pain

the "door"). If pain were as simple as a "visitor at the door," there would always be a clear pain generator and thus chronic pain would be rare. But, instead, chronic pain in the United States has grown from 50 million a few decades ago to 100 million today (Wells-Federman 1999; American Academy of Pain Medicine 2011). Pain would also not occur in limbs which are paralyzed or amputated if the Door Bell theory explained all pain nor would peripheral blocks fail to work.

Moreover, if pain were as simple as a "visitor at the door," fear, anger and anticipation of pain would not worsen pain as studies have clearly demonstrated. Cognitive Behavioral and relaxation therapies, psychological counseling and a change in attitude would not be so effective in reducing pain, as we reviewed in Chap. 4. Nor would antidepressant and antiseizure medications be effective in chronic pain if the pain were totally and only caused by a pain "visitor" at the door—a single pain generator.

Unlike unimodal, uncoordinated and "quick fix" pain treatment, multidisciplinary pain programs use a rehabilitation approach in which a "cure" for the pain or the underlying condition causing the pain is not the goal/aim. Rather the focus is on empowering patients and their families with knowledge and skills to improve function, decreasing the use of dependence-producing narcotics, providing physical and psychological skills and improving the quality of life of individuals with chronic pain, as seen in Table 8.1. Efforts are also made to return the patient to gainful employment where applicable.

During the golden age of chronic pain rehabilitation, Lipchik et al. found that "pain beliefs and attributions of pain control are amenable to change" with multidisciplinary treatment (Lipchik et al. 1993). The researchers found that patients' feelings of no control over their pain and tendency to cede control of their pain to medical professionals or family—two factors known to increase pain—diminished with even short-term multidisciplinary treatment which, in turn, "had a significant impact" on the patients' "subjective pain intensity." Patients given multidisciplinary care also "showed a reduction in the endorsement of the belief that their pain was an inexplicable mystery," reported the researchers (Lipchik et al. 1993).

Multidisciplinary treatment is also useful in getting the patient to decrease "pain behaviors" and replace them with "well behaviors." As we have noted in Chaps. 1–4, pain behaviors usually increase the subjective experience of pain; patients will often "feel" the way they act when they exhibit behavior like limping, signing, grimacing in pain and "guarding" against expected pain from normal activities. Pain behaviors can also stand in the way of the exercise and physical therapy which are almost always beneficial in chronic pain patients. *Until we educate patients, that "hurt" is not "harm" and that activity can be beneficial, patients will usually shy away from activities that would strengthen them and lessen their pain. Doing something which "hurts" so that "hurt" eventually becomes less, is certainly a counterintuitive concept and it is important that we convey it to our pain patients.*

"The psychology of the healthcare *provider* may be as important as the psychology of the patient," write Vranceanu et al. (2009). Clinicians may believe that biopsychosocial factors behind chronic pain are not within their domain, that they will "resolve after the nociception is addressed" or have an exaggerated belief in their own abilities to heal. They may also downplay biopsychosocial factors because of their stigmatization in society and/or believe that a patient's psychopathology is worse than it really is, declining involvement.

Clinicians can find patients with chronic pain "very frustrating" and worry that treating complex pain conditions will take too much time write Vranceanu et al. Some clinicians may use a "paternalistic model of decision making," encouraging a patient to be passive and denying him the chance to learn self-efficacy write the researchers. "A passive approach to treatment has been shown to increase disability and distress in many pain conditions." Clearly, all of these clinical "pitfalls" are highly unlikely with multidisciplinary care with its emphasis on biopsychosocial factors, team approach and encouragement of the patient's active participation in treatment. Even the family is encouraged to become active participants in multidisciplinary care, offering their opinions of what seems to work and what progress is being made.

Outcomes from Multidisciplinary Treatment

Studies of multidisciplinary pain programs, as we noted in previous chapters, have established positive outcomes, especially when compared to unimodal care. A 2003 study in *The Spine Journal* found that low back pain patients who completed a multidisciplinary rehabilitation program showed greater improvement on physical and mental measures and lost fewer days of work than those who received usual care (Lang et al. 2003).

A meta-analysis conducted by Flor et al. found patients treated with multidisciplinary care were twice as likely to return to work than untreated or unimodally treated patients and were functioning better than 75 % of those not treated with multidisciplinary care at follow-up (Flor et al. 1992). Multidisciplinary treatment was found superior to no treatment or unimodal treatment and benefits were

Table 8.2 Multidisciplinary outcomes estimates

Self-reported pain	Decreases by 30 %
Narcotic/opioid consumption	Decreases by 60 %
Physician visits for pain	Decreases by 60 %
Physical activity	Increases by 300 %
Gainful Employment	Increases by 60 %

Source: The role of the multidisciplinary pain clinic. Surgical Management of Pain, p. 87

maintained over a period of time, said the researchers—findings that they called "impressive." Both patients' subjective assessment of their pain and objective measures like return to work and usage of the healthcare system improved compared to groups not given multidisciplinary treatment.

On the basis of his own experience and published data Dr. Loeser estimates that patients who have completed multidisciplinary pain rehabilitation consume 60 % less opiates, visit medical professionals for pain 60 % less often and are 60 % more likely to return to work (Loeser 2014). Additionally, their physical activity increases by 300 % writes Dr. Loeser. Instituting follow-ups to multidisciplinary rehabilitation is important, adds Dr. Loeser, so patients retain these gains (Table 8.2).

Patients in a 2000 Denmark study enrolled in a multidisciplinary program did better than those in a general practice program on all instruments from pain to emotional state to quality of life to opioid consumption, writes Dr. Loeser. In fact, patients in the general practice group did not improve at all over a 6-month period while those in the multidisciplinary program did.

Multidisciplinary pain programs "offer the most efficacious and cost-effective, evidence-based treatment for persons with chronic pain," according to a 2006 *Journal of Pain* study Dr. Loeser quotes. "Unfortunately, such programs are not being taken advantage of because of short-sighted cost-containment policies of third-party payers" (Burchiel 2014).

Cantlupe writes in *Health Leaders* that as chronic pain impacts more Americans than diabetes, cancer and heart disease combined, hospitals, physicians, and health systems are seeking "integrative approaches to treat pain without narcotics" and that even the American Medical Association "has called for a multidisciplinary clinical approach to the treatment of chronic pain" (2013). As pain patients at Massachusetts General Hospital in Boston increased from 600 a month in 2007 to 1000 a month in 2013, the hospital increasingly moved away from unimodal and opioid treatments and made the services of psychologists, psychiatrists, and neurologists available, writes Cantlupe. After adopting a multidisciplinary care approach, Children's Hospitals and Clinics of Minnesota also reported positive results such as "savings and reduced lengths of stay" in children with pain said the *Health Leaders* article (Cantlupe 2013).

While "patient satisfaction" can suffer if patients do not receive the opioid medications they want or expect from providers, "patient attitudes about how hospitals control their pain is impacted by their perception of how the staff listens to them and cares about how they feel, with communication a key," says Michael Bottros, M.D., director of acute pain service at Barnes-Jewish Hospital and assistant professor of anesthesiology at the Washington University Pain Management Center.

In an article titled "What Has the Establishment of Multidisciplinary Pain Centers Done to the Improve the Management of Chronic Pain Conditions?" Howard Field, M.D. similarly notes cost, diagnostic, treatment and teaching advantages to a multidisciplinary approach to chronic pain (Fields 2011). Unimodal "procedurally oriented pain centers… offer primarily expensive care with less emphasis on rehabilitation and chronic care," writes Dr. Fields who founded the landmark Pain Management Center at the University of Southern California, San Francisco. A multidisciplinary approach is also superior to unimodal care in diagnosing "somatic pain and psychosocial problems," because of the volume of cases seen and provides an "optimal teaching environment," says Dr. Fields. Multidisciplinary treatment also offers Cognitive Behavioral therapy, physical therapy, vocational counseling and treatments often absent from unimodal care, notes Dr. Fields.

Dr. Loeser, while noting that patients in multidisciplinary programs tend to have more disability and psychopathology than other patients and there is an absence of outcome results for other treatment for these patients, believes multidisciplinary care is cost-effective. "Strieg et al. calculated that each patient treated in their pain clinic represented a savings of $280,000 in healthcare expenses until he or she reaches retirement age" (Loeser 2014).

Toward a "Virtual" Multidisciplinary Treatment for Patients with Chronic Pain

With the current lack of comprehensive multidisciplinary pain programs to address the complex needs of the patient with chronic pain, Primary Care Providers (PCP) including physicians, nurse practitioners, physician assistants and other clinicians are rightly frustrated. The referral to a "pain clinic" or "pain program" will usually result in unimodal treatments such as opioid prescriptions, epidural, facet and sac-roiliac injections, facet denervation (burning) or more expensive and controversial approaches like spinal cord stimulation (SCS) and Intrathecal Drug Delivery (IDD) systems, commonly known as morphine pumps.

In spite of everything the government and medical profession now recognize about opioid misuse, some of these "pain clinics" will place patients on high doses of opioids. Few will establish mutual goals with patients and send them to a physical therapist (PT), chiropractor or health psychologist. These establishments are much more likely to order X-rays, MRI scans and discograms despite the fact that pain generators seldom appear on such diagnostic tests but conditions that are *not* causing the pain *do* which risks over treatment. Such "pain clinics" are also notorious for telling patients to rest though, except for rare instances, activity is always better for chronic pain conditions. Thus, patients sent to these unimodally-oriented clinics often begin a downward spiral of more pain, more rest, more medications and more disability. These patients both risk becoming dependent on opioid medications and on the healthcare system itself.

How can you help your patients with chronic pain navigate through this morass to get control over their pain and their lives? Your first step, as your patient's advocate, is to focus on the "person" and not the "pain" and honor Hippocrates' words, "First Do No Harm."

Even providing a diagnosis for your patient without properly explaining all the aspects of it can be harmful. It is surprising to me how often physicians tell patients they have "damaged disks," a "pinched nerve/sciatica," "CRPS" (complex regional pain syndrome) or "fibromyalgia" without adding that the conditions are treatable, definitely manageable and do not need to cause significant disability. Too often physicians handing out such fearful diagnoses tell the patients only "what is wrong with them" and do not focus on what is "right with them"—the many aspects of their health that are just fine.

Certainly, there is often not adequate time in most practices to properly counsel a patient and his family about the origins and complexities of chronic pain and the many "dos and don'ts" (That is why I wrote a book to give to patients called *Pain: A Four-Letter Word You Can Live With* which is still in wide use). In the Internet age, this problem is compounded by the fact that a lot of readily available information about chronic pain is incomplete or incorrect. This is why on a patient's first visit, it is crucial to educate and empower him about the likely diagnosis, how it can be managed and what is "right" with a patient's health, to not unnecessarily alarm a patient.

For years, I have urged clinicians on my team, colleagues and students I teach to adopt the "Milwaukee" approach when advising a patient of a diagnosis, a methodology which is described in detail in the conclusion chapter of this book. As we explored in Chap. 3, a diagnosis or probable diagnosis, should be presented in terms of Milieu, Information, Label, Why, Aims, Understanding, Knowledge, Engagement of patient and End of visit—and re-presented this way at every subsequent visit. "Milwaukee" does not need to take too much time and the willingness to organize your thoughts and communicate information this way will empower your patient.

According to the American Pain Society, there are four types of patients who especially benefit from multidisciplinary treatment, as shown in Table 8.3 (Sanders 1995).

Patients with pathophysiological pain who are otherwise doing well

Patients with moderate-to-severe pathophysiological pain who cope poorly and are disabled (often with conditions like LBP and CRPS)

Patients with mild pathophysiological pain who cope poorly and are disabled (often with conditions like fibromyalgia or headache)

Patients with pain but no pathophysiology who may have psychological or substance use disorders

Table 8.3 Types of patients likely to benefit from multidisciplinary programs

Patients with pathophysiological pain who are otherwise doing well and need minimal reassurance
Patients with moderate-to-severe pathophysiological pain who cope poorly and are disabled (often with conditions like LBP and CRPS). These patients need an intensive focused multidisciplinary approach over several weeks
Patients with mild pathophysiological pain who cope poorly and are disabled (often with conditions like fibromyalgia or headache)
Patients with pain but no pathophysiology who may have psychological or substance use disorders. These patients may benefit not only from multidisciplinary care but also from long-term psychiatric and psychological care

How Do You Find Other Professionals to Develop the Virtual Team?

If you are a physician or primary medical provider, you need to know how to find the right therapist for your patient as well as other allied health professionals. Similarly, if you are a therapist or counselor/psychologist, you need to know how to find the right physician or primary care provider for your patient and others for a "team." Of course, not all physicians, physical therapists, occupational therapists and psychologists are the same even though they may have the same title and qualifications on paper. I recommend developing a checklist of professional qualities you seek in your virtual team members—including their location, hours and cost—and use it to develop a "stable" of clinicians that can be available to your patients. With trial and error and using feedback from your patients and other clinicians, you can identify the people who will strengthen your team.

Here are some guideline questions to ask as you assemble your team, shown in Table 8.4.

Does This Professional/Team Member

Respect and understand what I do?
Respect and cooperate with other disciplines?
Treat the "person" not "pain"?
Have a biopsychosocial approach?
Regard acute and chronic pain differently?
Have a favorable "bedside banner"?
Understand and use SMART goals? (discussed in this chapter)
Communicate with me in an accessible way?
Work towards the same goals that I am pursuing?
Suggest better ways of working with the patient?
Honestly advise when further treatment is unlikely to help patient?

Table 8.4 Qualities to Seek in a virtual multidisciplinary team member

Respect and understand what I do?
Respect and cooperate with other disciplines?
Treat the "person" not the "pain"?
Have a biopsychosocial approach?
Regard acute and chronic pain differently?
Have a favorable "bedside banner"?
Understand and use SMART goals? (discussed in this chapter)
Communicate with me in an accessible way?
Work towards the same goals that I am pursuing?
Suggest better ways of working with the patient?
Honestly advise when further treatment is unlikely to help patient?

An ideal pain program should offer both physical and psychological treatments including physical therapy, occupational therapy (OT), exercise, Transcutaneous Electrical Nerve Stimulation units (TENS), biofeedback, stress management, psychotherapy, nerve blocks, detoxification from addictive medications and education. It should monitor how well patients transfer their chronic pain management skills into their daily lives and include periodic follow-ups. Teaching effective pain management should be a program's focus, certainly not promises of a "cure." Especially effective in psychological treatment is the concept of "reframing"—helping the patient look at his situation differently although the facts are no different and cannot be changed. Psychological treatment can include relaxation training, problem solving, realistic goal setting, and several strategies described in Chap. 4, Cognitive Behavioral Treatment by Brad Grunert, Ph.D. and Kelly Smerz, Ph.D.

Objectives of a Multidisciplinary Pain Program

Multidisciplinary pain programs may be less plentiful than they were during their golden age but there is still widespread agreement about their goals, shown in Table 8.5. Even pain clinics and practitioners offering unimodal pain clinics and no multidisciplinary services, no doubt share some of the same goals for chronic pain patients though they may not be equipped to facilitate them (Sanders 1995).

1. Reduce the misuse of medication, especially opioids and benzodiazapines and invasive medical procedures
2. Maximize and maintain physical activity

Table 8.5 Goals of multidisciplinary treatment for pain

Reduce use of medication and invasive medical procedures
Maximize and maintain physical activity
Return patient to productive activity at home, work, and socially
Increase patient's self-efficacy, self-management, and self-care
Reduce subjective pain intensity
Improve patient's sleep and control depression
Reduce or eliminate use of healthcare system for primary pain care
Provide information for case settlements as needed
Minimize cost of treatment with no loss of quality
Induce an attitude of active participation in patient
Facilitate patient's better relationships with family and those at work
Encourage patient's maintenance of improvement with follow-up

3. Return patient to productive activity at home, work and socially
4. Increase patient's self-efficacy, self-management and self-care
5. Reduce subjective pain intensity, when possible
6. Improve patient's sleep and control depression
7. Reduce or eliminate patient's use of healthcare system for pain care
8. Provide information for case settlements as needed
9. Minimize cost of treatment with no loss of quality
10. Induce an attitude of active participation in patient (and family/friends)
11. Facilitate patient's better relationships with family and those at work
12. Encourage patient's maintenance of improvement with follow-up

Communication with Your Virtual Team

Certainly, in our current health car system, many providers cannot refer outside of their system—and insurance systems "lock" a patient to only seeing a certain group of providers. There are even significant penalties and copays for patients who seek care outside the system. However, some patients either have the flexibility or means to empower themselves and work through the system. Even if a multidisciplinary team is no longer under one roof (as it was during the golden age of multidisciplinary care) a "virtual" team can be assembled and achieve the efficient communication that Dr. Bonica sought over 60 years ago.

In a comprehensive pain center, such as the ones I have been involved in, a multidisciplinary team meets at regular intervals to discuss the status and progress of patients and make timely changes towards the mutually established goals. They are called "team conferences" or "staffing meeting". At all times patients are also present, sometimes with their family and case management nurses from the insurance company. As we have noted elsewhere in the "book, including a patient and his family in conferences about treatment and decision making is the hallmark of the multidisciplinary approach and differentiates it from unimodal" care.

Similarly, the patient, his family and the medical professionals on the virtual team can "meet" on a conference call or even through video conferencing. Even electronic mail has made it possible for all participants on a multidisciplinary care team to be in the "loop" about a patient's plan of care and progress, with appropriate safeguards for patient confidentiality and following HIPAA laws.

In addition to facilitating the coordination of care, sharing of goals and the input of different disciplines, there is another advantage to frequent virtual team conferences. If a patient is only interested in receiving opioids and passive treatments and not interested in being an active participant in care, this will be apparent when the team meets. Certainly passive treatments and opioid use tend to reinforce pain behaviors and the disability/illness conviction of the patient and can actually make treatment futile.

Who Are the Members of a Multidisciplinary Team?

Physicians, Other PCPs and Nurse Practitioners

To be useful on your team, these medical professionals which include limited license professionals, need to have a broad understanding of the biopsychosocial nature of pain and be able to obtain relevant history, perform examinations and prescribe appropriate medications. These potential team members need to be familiar with the many theories for pain perception outlined in Chap. 3 of this book and the pain behaviors they produce. These members need to believe the patient's report of pain yet refrain from excessive or unnecessary tests (avoiding the "X-ray diagnosis) and prescribing opioids.

The PCP should have a "function-oriented" treatment approach that focuses on the "person" and not the "pain" and be willing to work and receive input from other team members.

The focus of treatment should be on goal-oriented, time-limited treatment to empower patients to improve function. Appropriate antiseizure and antidepressant medications may be considered while opioids should *only* be used to enable a patient's participation in physical and psychological therapy prescribed and coordinated by the patient's primary care physician with appropriate documentation and following appropriate guidelines. One such recognized and recommended guideline is the Federation of State Medical Board's Model Policy on the Use of Opioid Analgesics in the Treatment of Chronic Pain (2013).

PCP should document their findings and share information with other team members within the limits of HIPPA law and assist patients with disability forms as needed. A PCP should rely on other medical consultants, especially those trained in chronic pain, in developing treatment such as psychiatrists, addictionologists (to titrate off opioids), interventional specialists (whose trigger point injections and other injections done in context of multimodal treatment can facilitate participation in therapy) physiatrists and other specialists.

Physical Therapist

The physical therapist is fundamental to a good multidisciplinary team. Rehabilitation of patients with pain, especially chronic pain, requires appropriate evaluation and aggressive activation with exercises. Not all physical therapists are trained or experienced in working with a broad understanding of functional improvement, however. Later in this chapter is a contribution from Nate Sorum, DPT, a doctorate in physical therapy and certified manual therapist who is a colleague of mine in Wisconsin.

Occupational Therapist

Occupational therapists help patients across the lifespan participate in all activities of daily living (ADL) such as dressing, washing, cooking, cleaning, hygiene, as well as in their work/occupations. Similar to physical therapists, occupational therapists focus on manual therapy for pain control and mobilization of joints to increase motion and function as well as body mechanics and proper posture as it relates to function and ergonomics. OTs are adept at creating splints, braces, and assistive/adaptive equipment fabricated to help perform activities safely. They also educate patients about joint protection techniques such as the use of larger joints in stable positions rather than small joints in unstable positions.

While some activities that OT direct may appear like "fun and games," they are graded activities to increase patients' range of motion, increase strength of muscles and endurance, improve posture and move toward SMART functional goals that are Specific, Measurable, Achievable, Realistic and Time-Based. They also educate patients about the benefits of activity versus inactivity and the important difference, while patients are active, between "hurt" and "harm."

In addition to helping patients acquire strength, stability and endurance in order to perform tasks at home or work, occupational therapists are skilled at helping patients with pain flare ups. OTs can help patients cope with these occasional periods of worsening of pain with the five "Ps": prioritizing, planning, pacing, positioning and problem solving that we explain in Chap. 6, Treating the Chronic Pain Patient.

OTs usually have a solid foundation in mind-body medicine and holistic treatment and are able to address the whole patient not just the "pain." In addition to helping adults decrease their disabilities and task specific inabilities, OTs can also specialize in problems of children, problems of the hand and in addressing the biopsychosocial needs of patients with chronic pain.

Psychologist and/or Trained Counselor

Psychologists and/or trained counselors are an essential part of any multidisciplinary team because of the interconnected biopsychosocial factors that contribute to complex chronic pain conditions. As we explored in Chaps. 1–4 of this book, stress, anger, resentment, and fear can exert huge effects on the chronic pain of patients, often without them realizing it. "Reframing" is an important concept for the patient to master, as well as other aspects of Cognitive Behavioral therapy. Isolation, loss of a vocation and social circle and feelings of being a victim or misunderstood also augment pain for many patients and the services of a psychologist or trained counselor are beneficial.

Other Multidisciplinary Team Members

In the current multidisciplinary program I work with, we retain a vocational counselor who is able to help patients seeking employment, including those with permanent restrictions resulting from injuries. Holding a master's degree, our vocational counselor also communicates with employers and insurance companies about a patient's progress and helps to coordinator the plan of care.

In previous programs, we have had a dedicated rehabilitation nurse who coordinates patient care and counseling. During the golden age of multidisciplinary rehabilitation programs and in some programs today, a breath of other specialists can be involved on the team such as a recreational therapist, biofeedback specialist, social worker, case manager, an ergonomics therapist, pharmacist, addictionologist, dietician/nutritionist and even clergy. Of course the patient and his family are also on the team. It has been said that in multidisciplinary treatment, "team" stands for Together Everyone Achieves More and my work over the decades continues to demonstrate the truth of this acronym.

The Role of the Physical Therapist on the Multidisciplinary Team

By *Nate Sorum, DPT*

The physical therapist plays a pivotal role on the multidisciplinary team. Charged with understanding both the underlying pathology of pain conditions, the psychosocial factors behind them and the kinesiology involved, the physical therapist not only treats pain but facilitates the patient's highest level of participation in ADL, including work where applicable, and therefore quality of life.

Traditionally, physical therapy has sought to improve patients' function and decrease pain by assisting in biomechanical changes to peripheral structures such as muscles, joints, fascia, ligaments and other tissues. However, the literature suggests that physical therapy interventions do more than merely affect the peripheral tissues—they also produce neurophysiological effects and influence central nervous system changes due to neuroplasticity. These neurophysiological effects modulates pain, neuromuscular control and psychosocial factors through complex central nervous system mechanisms, likely through the Matrix/Neuromatrix theory we explored in Chap. 2.

The multiple modes of physical therapy interventions, including education, movement, physical modalities like heat, cold and electrical stimulation and manual therapy, provide a breadth of treatments to improve the health and function of peripheral tissues at the same time as they facilitate adaptation in the central nervous system.

How Physical Therapy Works

Physical therapy aims to decrease functional limitations by deconstructing dysfunctional movements into discrete physical impairments such as decreased muscle strength, joint mobility and coordination. These deficits may be addressed independently or as part of a larger functional movement. Not every dysfunction may require intervention, but addressing the primary barriers is essential for optimal patient outcomes.

The physical therapist must continually reassess the emphasis on targeting specific biomechanical dysfunction versus general, aerobic conditioning and functional training to achieve the right balance. Pain, psychosocial factors, depression, anxiety, sleep quality, stress, coping, nutrition and medical pathology should be acknowledged and addressed by the physical therapist and other members of the multidisciplinary team because they can impact the success of reaching the physical therapy goals.

Physical therapy interventions can be classified into passive, active and educational. Passive treatments are performed *on* the patient, generally in early treatment, while active treatments are performed *by* the patient, starting with low intensity and increasing as treatment progresses. Educational interventions often focus on decreasing the fear of pain through the use of movement and emphasizing to the patient the difference between "hurt" (pain) versus "harm" (injury/ damage). By reassuring patients as they gradually increase their level of exercise with some controllable pain, they build confidence and increase their activities and their endurance towards mutually set goals.

Manual therapy and other passive treatments may make significant short-term changes, however long-term changes have not been shown (Gross et al. 2010). The patient's participation in active treatments, however, can create powerful long-term changes in the patient's functionality and pain.

Passive Treatments

Passive manual therapy interventions may include various techniques targeting soft-tissue, joint, or nerve mobility as well as neuromuscular function. Soft-tissue techniques may include myofascial release, strain-counterstrain, neurodynamic mobilization, massage, manual stretching, contract-relax stretching, instrument-assisted soft-tissue mobilization, manual trigger point release, active release technique and more. Joint-specific techniques include high-velocity, low-amplitude manipulation or graded mobilization and may also be used. Some physical therapy techniques such as muscle energy or functional mobilization treat both soft-tissue and joint restrictions, whichever is the most limiting. The primary aim of these varied treatments is to facilitate biomechanical movement, blood flow, tissue mobility and neuromuscular function as well as decrease nociception.

Some therapists offer "dry needling" which is thought to achieve a decrease in pain and muscle tonality through the elicitation of a local twitch response and has been used in the common complex pain conditions we reviewed in Chap. 10. Evidence of dry needling's effectiveness, however, is not persuasive and insurers are not likely to cover it (Dommerholt 2011).

Physical therapy modalities such as spinal traction, thermal modalities (hot/cold packs, diathermy, ultrasound), electrotherapy (TENS, IFC), and iontophoresis may be of short-term benefit but should not be used as primary interventions. They are useful in acute pain or a flare up of chronic pain, but only in conjunction with exercises and to facilitate improved function. Orthotics and splints may be used temporarily or permanently to facilitate mobility by compensating dysfunctional body regions.

Active Treatments

Active treatments such as therapeutic exercise, neuromuscular reeducation and gait training are major components of the overall treatment progression. Therapeutic exercise addresses specific strength, endurance, and mobility deficits which improve overall movement, improving functional activities and indirectly reducing pain perception. Neuromuscular reeducation includes addressing specific motor control/coordination/balance/postural/ body mechanics deficits, breathing pattern disorders, desensitization, mirror box and sensory discrimination training. These treatments may indirectly decrease pain by decreasing stress through certain body regions.

Aerobic conditioning is useful when incorporated into therapeutic exercise or gait training, but has *also* been shown to have a significant effect on pain in and of itself. Rainville et al. report, for example, that exercise programs improve behavior, cognition, affect and disability and global pain ratings in back pain syndromes (2004).

Recent research indicates that in addition to peripheral changes in the tissues, central nervous system modulation occurs with many of these physical therapy techniques (Bialosky et al. 2009). These central nervous system changes are described as neurophysiological effects such as modulation of nociception, muscle tone and descending pathways and neuromuscular changes (Delitto et al. 2012).

Educational Interventions

Education about positive or well behaviors including graded activity, graded exercise and the physiology of pain is always included in physical therapy treatments. Moseley et al. report that education about pain neurophysiology "changes pain cognitions and physical performance" and should be "included in a wider pain management approach" (Moseley et al. 2004). Physical therapists also may include education about stress, pacing, meditation, sleep hygiene, visualization, home exercise and self-management of symptoms based on their clinical experience and the needs of the patient.

Limitations of Physical Therapy

As discussed elsewhere in this book, there are two common mistakes made by physical therapists and other medical professionals. The first is regarding acute and chronic pain in the same way and using only the biomedical model which is rarely appropriate for chronic pain. The second is to attempt to treat complex pain problems within a limited scope of practice. Both of these mistakes can result in less than optimal outcomes and may be harmful to the patient's overall condition. Therefore physical therapists, whenever possible, should use the biopsychosocial model for treatment of a person suffering from chronic pain, and communicate with other providers treating their patient with chronic pain issues.

There is a fragile, but critical balance between treating tissue dysfunction and promoting independent management. Each patient deserves to be evaluated and treated by skilled and passionate healthcare professionals who can address the pathology, movement dysfunction, and psychosocial factors that may be present. However, when tissue dysfunction is labeled as the "pain generator" and the cause of their disability the patient can be harmed and made fearful. The patient may embark upon a lifelong search for the "cure" for his pain, perpetually seeking new practitioners.

Instead of seeking a medical "savior," patients should be focused on taking accountability for their condition and using different healthcare practitioners to guide them in their journey. No single healthcare practitioner can "fix" everything nor are all practitioners skillful but most healthcare practitioner can guide a patient in chronic pain down an empowered path of knowledge and independence.

If a patient with chronic pain hasn't shown significant functional improvement within 12 sessions, the current plan of care should be reexamined. "Chasing pain" is a risky game and results in poor patient satisfaction and unjustified healthcare costs. A high number of sessions may also facilitate a patient's dependency on passive treatments, as well as indicate poor functional improvement. After the patient has continued independently with a home exercise program for at least 6 weeks, an additional episode of care may be indicated which may include passive treatments. However the primary focus should not be on passive treatments but on advancing active treatments and reinforcing educational concepts. Realistic expectations and mutual goal setting are essential for a patient to feel that treatment has been beneficial and productive.

The ideal physical therapist should act more as a "trouble shooter" in collaboration with the patient than a "fixer" of dysfunction. The ultimate goal is to motivate the patient to take personal accountability for changing his physical condition through trust, rapport, empowerment, and encouragement while taking care to avoid a dependent relationship. Psychological techniques such as cognitive behavioral theory and motivational interviewing can be integrated with your physical therapy plan of care to facilitate lasting change in patient behavior upon completion of the treatment program.

Whether you are a physical therapist or work with one, you will provide the utmost benefit to your patients if you remember these truisms.

Each patient should be approached with confidence, humility, and flexibility.
Confidence is powered by experience, knowledge of research evidence, and best practices.
Humility is found in knowing one's limitations and the finite scope of your practice.
Flexibility is the ability to derive unconventional solutions to difficult problems to maximize the patient's quality of life.

Table 8.6 Main points of this chapter	
	Changed reimbursement patterns have decimated multidisciplinary programs
	Unimodal treatment overlooks behavioral, environmental, and societal factors
	Despite reimbursement patterns, you can set up a "virtual" multidisciplinary team
	"Team" members should be chosen on the basis of their philosophy and practice

References

American Academy of Pain Medicine. (2011). *Incidence of pain, as compared to major conditions.* Chicago: American Academy of Pain Medicine.

Bialosky, J. E., Bishop, M. D., Price, D. D., Robinson, M. E., & George, S. Z. (2009). The mechanisms of manual therapy in treatment of musculosketetal pain: A comprehensive model. *Manual Therapy, 14*(5), 531–538.

Bonica, J. (1990). Evolution and current status of pain programs. *Journal of Pain and Symptom Management, 5*(6), 368–374.

Burchiel, K. (Ed.), Surgical 708 management of pain. New York: Thieme.

Cantlupe, J. (2013, September). Confronting pain. *Health Leaders.*

Delitto, A., et al. (2012). Low back pain. *Journal of Orthopaedic and Sports Physical Therapy, 42*(4), A1–A57.

Dommerholt, J. (2011). Dry needling-peripheral and central sensitizations. *Journal of Manual and Manipulative Therapy, 19*(4), 223–237.

Fauber, J. (2015, January 12). Studies find little evidence of benefit from long-term opioid use. *Milwaukee Journal Sentinel.*

Federation of State Medical Boards. (2013). Model policy on the use of opioid analgesics in the treatment of chronic pain.

Fields, H. (2011). What has the establishment of multidisciplinary pain centers done to improve the management of chronic pain conditions? *Pain Management, 1*(1), 3–24.

Flor, H., Fydrich, T., & Turk, D. (1992). Efficacy of multidisciplinary pain treatment centers: A meta-analytic reviews. *Pain, 49,* 221–230.

Gross, A., et al. (2010). Manipulation or mobilisation for neck pain: A Cochrane Review. *Manual Therapy, 15*(4), 315–333.

Hanscom, D. (2012). *Back in control.* Seattle, WA: Vertus Press.

International Association for the Study of Pain. (2012). Interdisciplinary chronic pain management. *Pain: Clinical Updates, 20,* 7.

Lang, E., Liebig, K., Kastner, S., Neundorfer, B., & Heuschmann, P. (2003). Multidisciplinary rehabilitation versus usual care for chronic low back pain in the community; effects on life. *The Spine Journal, 3,* 270–276.

Leff, D. N. (1976). Management of chronic pain. *Medical World News, 18,* 54.

Lipchik, G., Milles, K., & Covington, E. (1993). The effects of multidisciplinary pain management treatment on locus of control and pain beliefs in chronic, non-terminal pain. *The Clinical Journal of Pain, 9*(99), 49–57.

Loeser, J. (2014). The role of the multidisciplinary pain clinic. In K. Burchiel (Ed.), *Surgical management of pain.* New York: Thieme.

Moseley, G. L., Nicholas, M. K., & Hodges, P. W. (2004). A randomized controlled trial of intensive neurophysiology education in chronic low back pain. *Clinical Journal of Pain, 20*(5), 324–330.

Rainville, R., Hartigan, C., Martinez, E., Limke, J., Jouve, C., & Finno, M. (2004). Exercise as a treatment for chronic low back pain. *The Spine Journal, 4*(1), 106–115.

Rosenquist, R. (2014). A hard lesson learned over two decades: Why specialists rarely use opioids for chronic pain. *Pain Consult.* Cleveland Clinic.

Sanders, S. (1995, July/August). Pain centers: What consumers want to know. *APS Bulletin,* p. 9.

Schatman, M. (2006). The demise of multidisciplinary pain management clinics? *Practical Pain Management, 6,* 30–42.

Vranceanu, A. M., Barsky, A., & Ring, D. (2009). Psychosocial aspects of disabling musculoskeletal pain. *The Journal of Bone and Joint Surgery, 91,* 2014–2018.

Wells-Federman, C. L. (1999). Care of the patient with chronic pain: Part I. *Clinical Excellence for Nurse Practitioners, 3*(4), 192–204; International Association for the Study of Pain (2012).

Chapter 9
Common Pain Problems: Low Back Pain

Low back pain (LBP), also called lower back pain and pain in the lower part of the spine, is the most common cause of disability in Americans under 45 (Wheeler et al. 2013). Defined as pain that occurs posteriorly in the region between the lower rib margin and proximal thighs, LBP sometimes unfortunately is called "back pain" which is a nebulous term that does not specify the "back" of what region. Unfortunately, the term is ingrained in medical and chiropractic terminology regardless of its imprecision.

LBP is the second most common chronic condition for which patients see a physician, fifth most common reason for hospitalization and third most common reason for surgery. According to the National Institute of Neurological Disorders and Stroke, LBP is also the most common cause of job-related disability" (2014). While not delving into all the complexities of LBP, this chapter provides my personal approach and philosophy of dealing with one of the most common pain problem seen by clinicians.

Chances are you have seen or will see patients with LBP. Its lifetime prevalence is 85 % and approximately 20 % of sufferers describe their pain as severe or disabling (Haldeman and Dagenais 2008). Aside from the indirect costs of LBP such as disability payments and loss of productivity, direct costs have been estimated at $12.2–$90.6 billion annually in the United States—comparable to the annual revenues of a Fortune 500 company like Toys "R" Us or Home Depot (Haldeman and Dagenais 2008).

In his comprehensive look at "Obamacare," *America's Bitter Pill*, Steven Brill observes that the United States spends $85.9 billion a year on back pain, more than it spends on state, county, and city/town police forces and that half of that expenditure is likely wasted (2015).

In spite of LBP's wide prevalence or perhaps *because* of it, there is significant controversy about its diagnosis and treatment. For example, over 200 treatments exist for LBP, yet many lack evidence-based research for their effectiveness leaving patients with frustrating outcomes and dependent on the healthcare system.

© Springer International Publishing Switzerland 2015
S. Vasudevan, *Multidisciplinary Management of Chronic Pain*,
DOI 10.1007/978-3-319-20322-5_9

There are numerous textbooks about LBP as well as self-help publications for the public, offering simplistic cures. Like most chronic pain conditions, many factors contribute to LBP and unimodal treatments are often ineffective.

LBP: Well Served by Multidisciplinary Rehabilitation Treatment

When it comes to LBP, there is "good news and bad news." The bad news is that in almost all cases, there is not an identifiable cause for the pain and diagnostic tests are not useful. The good news is that in about 90 % of the cases, patients will recover in a few months, *with or without* the wide variety of treatments currently available (Hazards 1994). Deyo and Weinstein report that 30–60 % of patients recover in 1 week, 60–90 % in 6 weeks, and 95 % recover from LBP in 12 weeks (Deyo and Weinstein 2001).

Clearly, conservative treatment and a "wait and see" attitude toward LBP is appropriate, approaches which are the foundation of multidisciplinary rehabilitation treatment. When Denmark implemented multidisciplinary care which included education, conservative treatment and "watchful waiting," it succeeded in cutting the rate of lumbar disk surgery in half in just 4 years (Rasmussen et al. 2005). "Between 1992 and 2001, the lumbar surgery rates in North Jutland County were reduced by approximately 50 %, with a steady downward trend," wrote researchers in *Spine*. "The reduction was even higher for elective first-time surgery."

In a *Journal of the American Medical Association* (JAMA) editorial Hadler et al. submit that LBP is overdiagnosed and overtreated, especially due to its financial relationship to workplace injuries (Hadler et al. 2007). "The back 'injury' construct holds that physical demands that render the pain less tolerable are the proximate cause of the back pain and hence the agent of 'injury,'" they write. Yet, back pain can no more be said to be "caused" by the workplace than the common cold, they contend.

Because of its huge costs to patients and employers in lost work time, researchers have sought predictors of LBP. In a JAMA article titled, "Will This Patient Develop Persistent Disabling Back Pain?," Chou and Shekelle present the case of a 48-year-old woman who has missed three work days due to LBP, has a history of chronic depression and is avoiding her usual activities and exercise and ask if she can be expected to develop "persistent disabling LBP" (Chou and Shekelle 2010). *Not surprisingly, the researchers conclude that a patient's tendency toward depression and fear and avoidance of regular activities can indeed predict that her LBP will become chronic or disabling.* The most helpful predictors, write Chou and Shekelle, are "maladaptive pain coping behaviors, nonorganic signs, functional impairment…and a presence of psychiatric comorbidities."

Vranceanu et al. have also examined the relationship between psychological states and disability from pain. "Research has established that a patient's attitudes, beliefs, expectations, and coping resources can increase or diminish pain intensity and pain-related disability," they write (2009). "Examples include misinterpretation or overinterpretation of pain as tissue damage rather than a temporary problem that will improve or a normal part of daily life, a belief that pain and disability will last forever (which leads to a passive, fatalistic approach to coping), and interpretation of pain as a sign of serious disease or a reminder of our mortality." The effect of emotional, cognitive, and psychological factors on pain is addressed in Chaps. 1, 2, 3, and 4 of this book.

As noted in those chapters, when we, as clinicians, reinforce patients' illness behaviors such as groaning, limping, sighing, and abandoning their activities of daily living, their pain can often worsen. Nor does uncoordinated, unimodal pain treatment help, as it still tends to focus on the "pain" and not the "person" say Vranceanu et al. "In spite of the strong support for the biopsychosocial model of illness, many providers persist in a strictly biomedical approach. They may believe that the illness dimensions they are seeing are not within their domain or that any psychosocial issues will resolve after the nociception is addressed. Even providers who do appreciate the psychosocial dimensions of illness may have difficulty addressing them because of the stigmatization of psychological illness in our society as well as an exaggerated belief in their own abilities to heal," write Vranceanu et al. (2009).

Multidisciplinary care is perceived by insurers and healthcare administrators to be more costly than unimodal care because of the team of medical professionals that may be deployed. But "costs may be offset by few lost wages or days off of work," write Chou et al. in a comparison of interventional therapies, surgery, and multidisciplinary rehabilitation for LBP in the journal *Spine* (2009a, b, c). Multidisciplinary care "is moderately superior" to unimodal care, write the researchers, in improving short- and long-term functional status and "the most effective programs generally involve cognitive/behavioral and supervised exercise components with at least several sessions a week, with over 100 total hours of treatment."

The persistence of unimodal treatments that are not evidence-based can be explained by the "intense competition by pharmaceutical companies, surgical instrument makers, and device manufacturers to convince stakeholders of the benefits of their products," says Haldeman and Dagenais (2008). "Only rarely do such promotional materials accurately present the scientific evidence underpinning a particular approach, and rarer still are discussions of potential harms." Haldeman lists 100 available and marketed treatments for LBP in the *Spine Journal*. Many and perhaps most lack an evidence base.

Epidural injections, for example, may help significantly in a few selected patients with nerve root irritation, but is overutilized, especially in patients with "chronic nonspecific LBP" write Chou et al. (2009a, b, c). The overuse of lumbar fusions and other surgeries despite the lack of evidence for their effectiveness, has produced a cohort of patients with failed back surgery syndrome (FBSS), write the researchers, a term for patients with persistent pain after they had surgeries, a condition rarely seen in countries other than the United States. In radiculopathy, epidural steroids decreased short-term pain compared to placebo; however, results were inconsistent and there were no effects on chronic pain or the need for surgery (Deyo and Chou 2014). Studies of injections for spinal stenosis associated with neurogenic claudication showed no benefits over placebo and the evidence for a benefit of epidural corticosteroids for axial back pain is sparse, say the researchers.

Even though he is a spine surgeon himself, David Hanscom, M.D., sees a broken healthcare system in the phenomenon of FBSS "a significant percentage" of which "could have been avoided with comprehensive rehabilitation" (Hanscom 2012). "In spite of my surgeon's bent-to-perform surgery, the most satisfying part of my practice is directing patients into a structured rehab program," he writes. LBP patients who received work hardening/work conditioning but not surgery had five times fewer physician visits than those who had surgery and they were half as likely to go on to have surgery reports Rogers et al. (2013). The diagnosis may be a "catch all" category, suggests the International Association for the Study of Pain's task force on pain in the workplace, noting that "fewer than 15 % of persons with back pain can be assigned to one of these categories of specific LBP" (Fordyce 1995).

Acute LBP Is a Back Attack©

As a physician treating pain conditions, many patients have told me that their backs had "gone out" but I never appreciated what a fearful experience it could be until it happened to me. More than a decade ago, after moving some furniture in the house, I found that the next day, I could not straighten up after getting out of bed. My back had "gone out."

Puzzled and a little alarmed I hobbled to work and soon realized I had to take the advice I had been giving to patients for years regarding conservative treatment. The "problem" resolved completely in 5–7 days. Still, episodes of back pain and stiffness and difficulty putting weight on my legs have recurred over the years, making me sympathetic to my pain patients and giving me a continual chance to "take my own advice."

For example, I have cautioned in this book about the dangers of the "X-ray diagnosis" and the very poor correlation between information shown on diagnostic imagery and the diagnosis and treatment of chronic pain. Like so many of my patients, the MRIs taken of my back when it "went out" revealed arthritis, "degenerative disk and facet joint arthritic changes" and spondylosis which are all normal for my age and were not the cause of the pain. They are physiologic changes that are part of aging and as normal and expected as grey hair.

As I counsel my patients, I quickly realized my lower back pain episodes could be prevented by lifestyle changes, regular exercise, losing weight, and stress management. Like my patients, I needed to practice self-management, self-efficacy, and self-care. By making a commitment to these practices I have been able to avoid injections, surgery, and drugs.

My own experience caused me to consider a new paradigm in understanding and educating patients about acute episodes of lower back pain. Sean Robinson, a medical student who did a senior rotation with me years ago, wrote a paper called "Back Attack: A New Paradigm" which well articulated the concept.

No one in the general population or the medical community fails to understand the concept of a heart attack—an acute episode of chest pain, associated with ischemia to the heart. Even when a heart attack is mild or does not require surgery, it is regarded as a sobering "wake-up call." Once stabilized, the physician will advise the patient to enact lifestyle changes like losing weight, exercising, eating better, decreasing cholesterol, decreasing stress and of course to cease smoking if he smokes. Risk factors for a future heart event like high blood pressure, diabetes, and increased cholesterol will be closely watched.

Yet a similar change in attitude and "wake-up call" doesn't happen with a back attack *even though a LBP episode is followed by additional episodes if no changes are made and the back attack is almost always a culmination of unhealthy life decisions*!

Of course, 1–5 % of patients who have a "back attack" may be experiencing fracture, progressive neurological problems like cauda equine syndrome, infection, cancer, visceral problems like pancreatitis and aneurysms which require quick and aggressive medical and possibly surgical treatment. But most "back attack" patients have no serious disease or condition and their pain will be self-limiting and resolve with time (Kinkade 2007). Studies on the natural history of back pain show that 30–60 % of patients recover in 1 week, 60–90 % recover in 6 weeks, and 95 % recover in 12 weeks. The bigger medical problem is relapses and recurrences which occur in about 40 % of patients within 6 months.

MacDonald et al. have suggested that a recurrence of LBP is linked to a change in patients' control of their back muscles, including both an absence of deep muscle back activity when returning to standing from full flexion (compared to controls) and an absence of normal back muscle relaxation at full trunk flexion (MacDonald et al. 2009). The former "would be expected to reduce the control, or fine-tuning of segmental motion associated with lumbar injuries," they write, while "the increased activity of superficial back muscles may serve to limit tensile forces and motion of injured/painful structures in the back." Even during remission, LBP patients with these alterations do not seem to return to normal anatomically write MacDonald et al.

Since the 1960s, cardiac rehabilitation has been the gold standard to prevent subsequent heart events. It encompasses multiple factors like graded mobilization, risk reduction, nutritional counseling for weight and lipid reduction, psychological and vocational counseling, smoking cessation, stress reduction and self-responsibility. Cardiac rehabilitation team members have included physicians, cardiologists, therapists, nurses, nutritionists, and psychologists.

The same multifactorial approach should be routinely employed for "back attacks" for the same reasons; if a patient continues to live in the same way, he risks the same medical events. Herta Flor, a neuroscientist and the scientific director of the department of Neuropsychology at the University of Heidelberg, has written extensively about the efficacy of multidisciplinary pain programs after acute pain events. Because of the role of learning and memory processes in the development and maintenance of chronic pain and the possibilities created by the brain's plasticity, multidisciplinary treatment is particularly effective she says (2015). The value of a multidisciplinary team is further explored as a resource by Dr. Flor and Dennis Turk, M.D. in *Pain: An Integrated Bio-Behavioral Approach* (2011).

In the case of my own "back attack" and multitudes of patients who sustain them, there is little rationale to obtain X-rays or other diagnostic imagery unless red flags are present (Haswell et al. 2008) Conservative treatment with 1–2 days of bed rest, followed by reactivation, medications, and thermal modalities (cold/heat) for comfort and physical therapy over a period of 2–6 weeks, are sufficient (Deyo and Weinstein 2001; Patel and Ogle 2000).

When patients are taught the difference between "hurt" and "harm," self-responsibility and self-efficacy, and encouraged to resume activities soon, studies show they have less pain, improved functional status and miss less work (Deyo and Weinstein 2001). It is important, though, that you counsel your patients to avoid heavy lifting, repetitive bending, twisting, and prolonged sitting when they resume their activities after acute LBP.

Just as the American Association of Cardiovascular and Pulmonary Rehabilitation (AACVPR) recognizes the importance of physical, psychological, and social changes in reducing death and disability from a heart attack, the COST B13 Working Group has established "European guidelines for the management of chronic nonspecific LBP" (AACVPR 2015; Airaksinen et al. 2006). Similarly, core strengthening and other exercises specifically for LBP can prevent a recurrence such as McKenzie exercises (McKenzie 1980).

I believe a back pain paradigm based on the heart attack paradigm can help the millions affected by repeated episodes of lower back pain in understanding their condition and susceptibilities and preventing further "back attacks." Rather than "medicalizing" an attack of LBP or Back Attack, this new paradigm would help patients avoid the current odyssey of multiple surgeries, injections, and chronic opioid use—which only worsens pain as it adds to health care and societal costs.

Common Causes of LBP

There are many factors that contribute to LBP though few can be pinpointed in diagnostic imagery or laboratory tests. Here are some common causes of this frequent condition which are highlighted in Table 9.1.

Table 9.1 Leading causes of back pain

Soft tissue problems	Posture, muscle strain, ligament sprains
Bone and joint conditions	Fracture, osteomyelitis, tumor or arthritis
Discogenic conditions	Herniation, foraminal or spinal stenosis
Infection	Discitis and osteomyelitis
Other causes	Stress, inflammation, circulation problems

Soft Tissue Problems

Problems with the muscles and ligaments in the lower back are the most frequent cause of LBP. Poor posture, muscle strain and ligament sprains from work-related injuries, motor vehicle accidents, or sports injuries are the biggest triggers in patients. Pain associated with such tissue-related LBP overlaps with myofascial pain, discussed in the following chapter (along with fibromyalgia and complex regional pain syndrome). Guidelines from the American Pain Society recommend that problems with the muscles and ligaments in the lower back be termed "nonspecific LBP" (Chou et al. 2007).

Bone and Joint Conditions

LBP can be caused by a fracture or dislocation of the spinal column from injury, osteomyelitis, tumors of the bone or arthritis of the facet joints. Clinicians must always weigh these possibilities when first examining a patient. Congenital causes of LBP, such as patients who were born with abnormally developed bones in the lower back, represent a very small percent of patients with bone and joint-caused LBP.

Discogenic Conditions

The lumbar disks are also a common cause of LBP. Often a patient's nucleus pulposus, the gel-like material enclosed in the annulus fibrosis that acts as a cushion between the bones in the vertebrae, has broken out through a weakness in the outer annulus and caused a herniation of the disk. Herniation of a disk is more common in young patients, between the ages of 20 and 45 and may happen acutely when the patient has lifted and twisted at the same time, placing excessive force on the disk, though it can occur spontaneously with no injury. MRI scans of asymptomatic patients often show "disk bulge" or "disk herniation," common occurrences.

Herniation is less likely in older patients because the lumbar disks become dry as a person ages. However, older patients may instead present with foraminal stenosis and spinal stenosis because disks tend to degenerate with age, causing disk space narrowing and setting up a cascade that produces degeneration of facet joints, leading to degenerative disk disease/facet arthritis, generally referred to as lumbar spondylosis.

As we have noted, there is a very poor correlation between pain experienced by patients and "pain" explanations revealed on MRIs and other diagnostic imagery (Groopman 2007). And there is another drawback to diagnostic imagery: it often reveals "problems" in asymptomatic patients putting them at risk of unnecessary care for conditions that would never have caused pain and seldom pinpoints the source of pain in patients who *are* symptomatic. Unnecessary and excessive diagnostic films raise healthcare costs. They are most beneficial when clinicians are trying to rule out "red flags" that could require immediate medical or surgical treatment.

In 1934, two US surgeons described how LBP and leg pain could be relieved through removal of a disk and since that time, the diagnosis of disk-related back problems has been a cornerstone of many pain and orthopedic practices (Mixter and Barr 1934). However, most experts now agree that less than 5 % of all patients with disk-related back pain require surgery. Most discomfort can be managed with the educational and conservative approach that characterizes multidisciplinary treatment.

Infection

Almost half of patients receiving surgery for disk herniation were infected with the gram-positive human skin commensal Propionibacterium acnes reported researchers from the University of Southern Denmark and the University of Birmingham, England in the *European Spine Journal* (Nordqvist 2013). In a companion study, pain and disability in patients with LBP given the antibiotic amoxicillan and clavulanate for 100 days diminished. "The study is very interesting and…supports the hypothesis of infectious discitis causing 'degenerative' disk disease. It may also explain why ozone therapy helps back pain because ozone is an effective antimicrobial agent," remarked Dr. Solsberg, a neuroradiologist and interventional pain physician in Englewood, CO.

Other Causes

Sometimes LBP is not related to activity at all but results from day-to-day stress. The same daily tension that might manifest as a tension headache in one patient may manifest as LBP in another. Thus LBP might be considered a "tension headache" of the spine and has been referred to as "tension myalgia" by John Sarno (1984). Luckily, multidisciplinary treatment is usually effective in teasing out pain which is driven by stress factors.

There are other times when LBP is linked to inflammation of pelvic organs such as the uterus or indicates the presence of a kidney stone. Circulation problems such as an aortic aneurysm can also cause LBP, so obviously treatment of LBP should always start with a thorough examination.

Diagnosis of Back Pain

The diagnosis of LBP is based on a review of a detailed patient history and an examination by a physician. Included in the diagnosis should be the type of pain, how and when it started, if related numbness and tingling are present, and whether the pain is associated with a particular activity. A physical examination should check for muscle spasm, trigger points, decreased motion of the spine, muscle weakness, and neurological signs such as alteration in reflexes, decreased sensation, and weakness of specific muscles.

X-rays are appropriate to ascertain that there is no fracture, tumor or arthritis, but will rarely help you verify patient's pain or pinpoint its cause. In cases in which sciatica or herniation have been established, a CAT scan or MRI may be valuable in determining facet disease or nerve compression. Rarely, a myelogram, using an injected dye, is used to localize a problem but CAT scans and MRIs have largely replaced myelograms.

Another test which can be valuable in some cases is the electromyogram (EMG) which identifies the presence, level, and degrees of nerve compression. The EMG can also identify any general nerve or muscle disease contributing to the pain. It is usually performed by a specialist in Physical Medicine and Rehabilitation or neurology.

Smoking and Low Back Pain/Chronic Pain

An estimated one-in-five adults in the United States uses tobacco everyday or some days, which equates to 50 million people and 21.3 % of the overall population (Frellick 2014). Smoking is more common in men (26.2 %) than women (15.4 %) and is most common among adults 25–44 years (25.2 %). Interestingly, the prevalence of tobacco use is nearly twofold higher in patients with chronic pain and making it an issue of clinical importance to your practice (Ditre et al. 2013; Ekholm et al. 2009).

In a recent review titled "Updates on Smoking and LBP" Shanti and Shanti note that although nicotine has analgesic properties, over time, it alters pain processing and contributes to the development of chronic pain and greater pain intensity (2014). While referencing 57 related papers, the authors note the following as also shown in Table 9.2.

1. Nicotine is an agonist of acetylcholine receptors found throughout the peripheral and central nervous system; these in turn release neurotransmitters such as dopamine and the mesolimbic reward system, reinforcing nicotine use.
2. The anti-nociceptive effects of nicotine also may be mediated by activation of the endogenous opioid system.

Table 9.2 Putative pain actions of nicotine

Acetylcholine receptors	May activate dopamine and mesolimbic reward system
Anti-nociceptive effects	May activate endogenous opioid system
Neuroendocrine and HPA effects	Blunt pain perception and stress response
Analgesic effect	May derive from presser effect
Analgesic effect	May derive from 5HT, NE, GABA activity; suppression of inflammation or evoked potentials, attention narrowing

3. Smoking causes changes in the neuroendocrine system that could modulate pain perception and there is blunting of the "stress response" by affecting hypothalamic-pituitary-adrenal (HPA) activation.
4. The pressor actions on the cardiovascular system have been hypothesized to play a role in the analgesic effect of nicotine.
5. Other proposed mechanisms for the analgesic effects of nicotine include: attentional narrowing, release of norepinephrine and serotonin, gamma amino butyric acid (GABA) receptor activity, regulation of inflammatory response, and suppression of pain-related evoked potentials.

Ekholm et al. found that "cigarette smoking was significantly increased in individuals suffering from chronic pain and in opioid users, smoking was further increased" (2009). In a review article Shanti and Shanti write that "The data suggested a positive correlation between the smoking dose and risk of LBP" and that "smoking was linked to an increased risk of transitioning from sub-acute back pain to chronic back pain."

The authors also note "In addition to altering pain processing, smoking can contribute to structural changes that may increase the risk of chronic pain conditions. For example, smokers are at increased risk for osteoporosis, fracture, lumbar disk disease, impaired wound healing, muscular damage, and impaired healing from spinal fusion, possibly because of impaired oxygen delivery to tissues and accelerated degenerative process."

Weingarten et al. reviewed the association between smoking status, pain intensity, and functional interference in patients with chronic pain and note that cigarette smoking may be associated with painful musculoskeletal disorders, use of more analgesic medication than non-smokers, and more back pain and functional limitations than non-smokers and concluded that "current smokers reported significantly greater pain intensity and pain interference with functioning. Symptoms were more pronounced in smokers with more severe nicotine dependence" (2008). *Thus, it is important for physicians and every clinician to provide education and resources to help patients with chronic pain, especially lower back pain, quit smoking.*

Treatment of Back Pain

Anyone who has watched late night TV, between midnight and 5 a.m. (like I do when I am working on projects or patients with chronic pain, because they cannot sleep), sees commercials and infomercials touting braces, electrical devices, traction, herbal products, shoe inserts, exercise balls, special shoes, special mattresses, calf bands, and numerous other products that are "guaranteed to relieve pain or eliminate pain, especially LBP." Like my patients, I wish it were true! Unfortunately, there is no such cure-all or panacea for the complexities of LBP.

Table 9.3 Treatments for low back pain

Treatment	Key points
Rest	A few days, not weeks
Medication	Avoid opioids and benzodiazepines long-term
Exercise	Beneficial as it is in all chronic pain
Back protection	Useful techniques can prevent harm
Surgery	Sometimes necessary though often, not
Ergonomics	Workplace modifications often possible
Injections	Epidural and trigger point injections in selected patients early
Manipulation	Physical therapists, chiropractors, self-care
Electrical stimulation	TENS units allow patients to self-manage
Temperature modalities	Cold followed by heat often effective
Biopsychosocial factors	Multidisciplinary care
Brace/supports traction	Older, mechanical methods with little evidence-based studies
Education	Useful techniques can prevent harm

What we as clinicians need to do is help the patient understand the multifactorial nature of LBP and learn appropriate lifestyle modifications and exercises, after we rule out "red flags" that would suggest a more serious condition.

Despite over 200 different treatment approaches described for treating lower back pain, very few are evidence-based. Yet, these treatments, especially invasive, unimodal ones, are often chosen by patients, clinicians, and third-party payers, because they are widely publicized and advertised. The problem is they usually produced outcomes that are no more favorable than conservative treatment. This is dismaying because in up to *90 % of patients with acute LBP*, *their pain will resolve, irrespective of the treatment* that is given within a period of days or weeks (Hazards 1994).

Table 9.3 shows the many treatments for LBP which include, but are not limited to, surgery.

Rest

We have talked a lot in this book about the value of chronic pain patients staying active and avoiding excessive rest. In the acute phase of LBP, there is a qualification: rest is valuable because it decreases gravity pulling on the spine. Still, the length of rest time that we recommend has shortened from the 1980s when 2–3 weeks were recommended to today when 3–4 days are considered sufficient. During the first few weeks, a patient recovering from acute LBP should avoid strenuous or heavy work, however (Hegmann 2007).

Medication

As we saw in Chap. 6, Treating the Chronic Pain Patient, there are many medications that can be helpful in chronic pain. The first category includes anti-inflammatory medications like aspirin and ibuprofen (NSAIDs or nonsteroidal anti-inflammatory drugs) and cortisone. Used for 2–3 weeks, these medications decrease both the pain and inflammation of LBP. Tylenol can also be useful though it lacks the anti-inflammatory actions of aspirin and ibuprofen. Another category of medicines that can be helpful are muscle relaxants such as cyclobenzaprine (Flexeril), Metaxalone (Skelaxin), tizanidine (Zanaflex), or Baclofen (Lioresal). Conversely, benzodiazepines like Valium and opioids such as oxycodone/OxyContin should be given with great caution for LBP because of their abuse potential. Their use should be limited to a few days or weeks in conjunction with active mobility or therapy such as physical therapy or chiropractic care.

Temperature Modalities

In the first 72 h after the onset of back pain or LBP, cold is an effective treatment applied locally. Thereafter, heat, applied locally three to four times a day, can produce pain relief, muscle relaxation, and a decrease in spasms. Applied heat also decreases stiffness and prepares muscles for stretching. Deeper heating modalities such as ultrasound, used in conjunction with physical therapy for six to eight sessions, can be used to provide relief to patients. Heat modalities break the "pain-tightness-pain" cycle which can perpetuate pain.

Exercise

For decades excellent exercises have existed that address the muscles involved in LBP. In 1950, Paul Williams, M.D., described a series of exercises that strengthened the buttocks and abdominal muscles while stretching the muscles of the lower back and the hamstrings. Subsequently, the McKenzie exercises were popularized for LBP and remain in wide use. In 2010, Norman Marcus, M.D. published the best-selling, *End Back Pain Forever* which also demonstrates effective exercises for LBP. None of these exercises have been shown to be superior to others (2012). My personal recommendation is for patients to practice the Williams flexion and McKenzie extension exercises and a program of "lumbar stabilization" exercises that strengthen "core muscles" while stretching tight muscles. I believe Dr. Marcus' exercises are also worthwhile and his book is a good resource for patients with LBP, especially when it persists beyond several months. Yoga, Pilates, and "core conditioning" are also beneficial exercises. General conditioning, aerobic and flexibility exercises will prevent frequent or recurrent flare ups of LBP.

Back Protection/Education

Probably the single most important change for patients with LBP is to learn to practice appropriate lifting and to understand the effects of back posture on pain. Specifically, patients need to learn to carry objects close to their body rather than held out at arm's length. Patients should be educated to use the strong muscles in the leg for lifting rather than back muscles, which will decrease stress on the spinal column. Common sense techniques such as pushing rather than pulling an object, using foot rests and using step stools for overhead reaching are also proven to reduce LBP. It is no surprise that good health habits also exert a positive effect on LBP such as weight reduction through diet and exercise, general physical conditioning and flexibility and avoiding the use of tobacco. While most physical therapists can guide your patients in these simple and effective techniques, formal educational programs, sometimes called "back schools," are also available.

Surgery

When there is clear evidence of a disk herniation causing compression of a nerve, surgery is necessary. In these cases, removing the pressure on the nerve substantially removes leg pain and prevents further neurological deterioration. Surgery is also appropriate when there is some instability of the spine and a fusion of the vertebrae is usually performed. Sometimes a patient will develop cauda equina syndrome, a situation in which a disk has herniated backwards. Characterized by sudden weakness in both legs and loss of bladder and bowel control, cauda equina syndrome is considered an emergency and requires prompt surgery to remove the pressure on the nerves.

While surgery is necessary in these cases, it is important to note that there is little evidence of effectiveness of spinal fusion on LBP despite its popularity as a surgical intervention. "No subset of patients with chronic LBP could be identified for whom spinal fusion is a predictable and effective treatment," write Willems et al. (2013).

It is beyond the scope of this book to address surgery for LBP in depth but both clinicians and patients need to exercise caution when considering surgery as the first choice. From the hospital profiteering chronicled in Steven Brill's *America's Bitter Pill* and Jerome Groopman's *How Doctors Think*, to the back injury "franchise" described by Nortin Hadler in *Stabbed in the Back* and John Sarno's *Mind Over Back*, much back surgery seems to do more for the health of *providers* than patients (Brill 2015; Groopman 2007; Hadler 2009; Sarno 1984). Kim J. Burchiel, M.D., editor of *Surgical Management of Pain* (2014) writes, "In the case of spine surgery, *more* care is not clearly predictive of *better* care."

While the Spine Patient Outcomes Research Trial (SPORT) studies concluded that discectomy at single level in selected patients with clear disk herniation and radiculopathy was associated with improvement, surgery should be a *mutual decision between the patient and his surgeon.*

Of all medical treatment, surgery no doubt poses the most risk and expense so patients must be able to weigh the evidence. The goal of shared decision-making is to educate the patient about the surgeries' "trade-offs and uncertainties, so that the patient can make decisions consistent with his preferences, values and goals," says an American Pain Society Clinical Guideline (2009). "Formal shared decision-making aids have been shown to decrease the proportion of patients who choose spine surgery, without adversely affecting clinical outcomes."

Nerve Blocks/Trigger Point Injections

Injection of anesthetics and/or cortisone around inflamed or irritated nerves can be helpful in decreasing leg pain associated with disk herniation. The procedures, usually called epidural blocks, are sometimes performed by anesthesiologists, depending on the degree of discomfort a patient is experiencing. Chou et al. in an American Pain Society Clinical Practice Guideline however have written that despite the increase of epidurals by 271 % and facet joint injections by 231 % in the 1990s, "increased utilization of interventional therapies and surgeries has not been associated with improved health status among patients with LBP and may be one factor contributing to increases in healthcare expenditures associated with back pain" (2009a, b, c). Moreover, Jarvik et al. report that "Epidural steroid injections do not offer any substantial advantage over lidocaine."

Deyo and Chou write that "there is no high quality evidence that trigger point injections are effective for back pain" and "their role in chronic back pain should be limited (if used at all), and only after alternatives fail" (2014).

Patients who continue to experience pain accompanied by significant radiation of pain to the legs and buttocks after an injury or surgery on the lower back are sometimes treated with trigger point injections. Trigger points are hyperirritable, tender spots in a muscle that produce pain and other symptoms like tingling and numbness far away from the spots themselves. An injection of anesthetic and/or cortisone followed by stretching has been found to help patients, especially when combined with education and support from a multidisciplinary team.

Electrical Stimulation

Transcutaneous Electrical Nerve Stimulation (TENS) is widely used in patients with LBP, especially with accompanying sciatica/pain running down the leg. It is particularly useful when there is clear evidence of nerve compression. Electrical stimulation treatment also has the advantage of encouraging self-efficacy in patients since it is a modality they apply themselves.

Stimulation of the spinal cord was first described in the 1950s as Dorsal Column Stimulation but the procedure was abandoned because of the extensive surgery required. More recently, newer technology allows fine electrodes to be placed over the spinal cord, through the skin, thereby providing for selective stimulation along the back. For patients who have received no relief from other pain reduction methods and who have significant scarring around a nerve, TENS units can reduce pain and improve function. They can lead to increased function and a reduction in pain medications. In my personal experience, 5–10 % of patients get relief from TENS units.

Ergonomics

Ergonomics is the science of making jobs in the workplace fit the people who perform them to lessen muscle fatigue, increase productivity, and reduce the number and severity of work-related injuries. Adjustable workbenches, adaptable chairs, and other alterations that decrease bending, stooping, and twisting activities of the spine are examples of ergonomics that can reduce back pain. When a job activity or environmental condition cannot be modified, a patient can be taught how to do the same job in a more efficient manner through the proper body mechanic training. Unimodal and uncoordinated chronic pain treatments rarely included ergonomics but they are a cornerstone of multidisciplinary treatment and another reason for its positive outcomes.

Manipulation

Manipulation involves the use of the hands to distract the tissues of the lower back. When done gently by physical therapists, manipulation is often referred to as mobilization. Doctors of chiropractic medicine frequently perform such manipulations and refer to them as adjustments. Manipulation is often readily embraced by patients because it is simpler and more "natural"—avoiding medications and injections— and often feels good. Patients can also be taught to perform some stretching and mobilization techniques on themselves and are encouraged to do so, after six to eight sessions with a professional. Self-manipulation is another example of self-efficacy and self-management that helps chronic pain patients avoid dependency on the healthcare system and on medications.

Brace/Supports Traction

In the past, corsets and braces were used to support the lower back and thus relieve pain. The devices served as a warning to wearers to be careful with bending and lifting activities and were more of a reminder than a "cure." They also relieved pressure on lumbar disks by increasing pressure on the abdomen. However, these supporting devices have fallen out of favor as more effective modalities have become available. Similarly, traction—pulling the parts of the body apart through force— has fallen in popularity. While traction for neck pain can be effective, traction for LBP has not particularly been effective.

Biopsychosocial Factors

A few years ago, research was presented at a meeting of the American Academy of Pain Medicine that revealed how potent a force fear can be in pain patients. In a study conducted at Stanford University, Sean Mackey, M.D., Ph.D., Chief of the Pain Management found that "Those who had more fear during an acute LBP episode were much more likely to ultimately overpredict the amount of pain they had, which ultimately led to significant increase in fear-avoidance behaviors, with subsequent worsening of symptoms, increase in duration of pain, and increase in disability" (Frieden 2011).

In Chaps. 1, 2, and 3, we looked at the complex biopsychosocial factors that contribute to chronic pain including the role of fear. Pain that patients think is normal, such as pain after exercise, does not generally produce the anticipatory pain and fear we see in chronic pain when a patient thinks the sensations are "harmful."

Treating the Patient with Low Back Pain

Once a physical evaluation and history have been taken of a patient's LBP, there is a "cafeteria" of noninvasive treatment approaches available as we see in Table 9.4. Because, LBP will generally improve over time, regardless of the treatments given, a conservative, "wait and see" approach is prudent, assuming acute situations that require surgery have been ruled out. Often this means reassuring the patient and giving him simple guidelines for taking responsibility for his own LBP.

Table 9.4 General low back pain advice for patients

Activity
Weight control
Stop smoking
Stretching
Correct posture
Exercise
Stop unnecessary medication

Activity

While a few days, usually two, of rest are desirable to remove pressure on the spine, prolonged bed rest actually increases the stiffness and pain in patients with LBP (Deyo and Weinstein 2001). Conversely, physical activity decreases inflammation, muscle tightness and tension, allowing better blood flow and nutrients to diffuse. As seen in almost all chronic pain conditions, exercise greatly assists in recovery and decreases pain. Activity also has strong psychological benefits, increasing feelings of self-efficacy and distracting focus on pain.

Weight Control

While I have seen many thin patients who still have LBP and many obese patients who do not, being overweight is often linked to LBP. There is clear evidence that every pound of weight that a patient loses decreases 3–4 lb of pressure on the spine, joints of the hips, knees, and ankles. When patients stay within 10 lb of their ideal weight, pain is usually controlled or absent. It is important for you to motivate your LBP patients to keep their weight under control by giving support and encouragement and connecting them with resources such as fitness programs when feasible. Patients who overeat often suffer from low self-esteem so positive messages are preferable to criticism. The positive effects from exercise also improve patients' self-esteems and keep them motivated to continue with diet and exercise programs.

Stop Smoking

As we discussed earlier, for general health reasons, no patient should be smoking cigarettes—ever! But studies demonstrate that nicotine particularly causes or worsens back pain by restricting blood flow to muscles and disks themselves. As we noted earlier in this chapter, smoking is very prevalent in chronic pain patients and is seen to worsen their pain through deleterious effects on several systems. Patients who smoke also do extremely poor after fusion surgery (2014). As with overweight and obesity, it is better to offer patients positive messages about how they can quit smoking than criticism.

Correct Posture

Advice to prevent or control LBP during activities of daily living is readily available to patients from physical and occupational therapists, ergonomic and vocational experts and from the "back schools" we mentioned earlier. There are also many books that address ways to keep from aggravating LBP and even online advice. Patients are told to use appropriate posture during all activities including a back cushion to maintain curvature of the back while driving. While sitting, patients are advised to prop their feet on a stool to keep at least one knee and if possible both knees higher than the hip. Sitting for over 30–45 min should be avoided in general as this can cause increased pressure on the disk and tightness of the muscles. Patients should get up and move around. Some workplaces have even instituted "stand desks" to help workers minimize the harmful effects of too much sitting.

Stretching

Stretching may be the most important exercise for LBP. The value of stretching is encapsulated in the saying "a long muscle is a strong muscle" and it is why you frequently see sports figures stretching whether they are playing baseball, basketball or another sport. Many exercise programs incorporate stretching, including, of course, yoga but make sure to caution your patients not to stretch past their limits. A stretch should be "slow, steady, and sustained" and stopped if it hurts. "Bouncy" stretches, frequently described as ballistic stretches, are not useful for LBP.

The second most valuable exercise for back pain after stretching is aerobic conditioning exercises such as walking, bicycling, and dancing—anything that gets the heart pumping and makes someone perspire. Walking is probably the easiest and most realistic exercise for patients but if a patient has significant arthritis of the knees and hips, a stationary bicycle might be more appropriate. Swimming is an optimal exercise for patients who enjoy it. The trick is to find an exercise the patient enjoys so he will keep doing it.

During exercise and even when a patient is not exercising, it is worthwhile to encourage "deep breathing." Deep breaths improve oxygen flow to the muscles and promote relaxation, as we saw in Chap. 4 about Cognitive Behavioral therapy. Conversely, shallow, stressful breaths make pain and anxiety worse which is why patients are often told "don't forget to breathe." Also, when a patient expects pain and has anticipatory fear, his breathing will automatically become more shallow and rapid, which in turn, can increase pain sensations.

Other exercises that are useful for LBP patients are known as "core strengthening" exercises. They refer to the abdominal muscle in the front of the spine and the important muscles in the back that support the spine.

Strengthening exercises for LBP have undergone several pendulum swings over the last 50 years. Once, it was believed that strengthening only the abdominal muscles—the so-called Williams exercises—was necessary. Then "extension exercises" in which patients laid on their stomachs to strengthen the back muscles—the so-called McKenzie exercises—became popular. The goal of McKenzie therapy is to centralize the patient's pain in the core back structures rather than treat pain that is localized in a specific area such as the lower right posterior back or hip joint (McKenzie 1980). Patients doing McKenzie exercises may minimize or abolish their localized pain and achieve centralization over the course of daily exercises.

More recently, the core strengthening Pilates exercises have attracted followers. Most well-trained exercise therapists will combine the best of all these therapies for use in strengthening muscle groups.

Table 9.5 Main points of this chapter	LBP—one of the most common chronic pain conditions
	Conservative/multidisciplinary care is best
	LBP should be regarded as a heart attack—call for health and lifestyle changes
	Activity/exercise, not medications, most beneficial

Avoid Unnecessary Medication

We have discussed in many places in this book the limitations of opioid medications. Throughout much of the 1990s and 2000s, the medical profession erroneously believed opioid painkillers were less addictive than they really are and they were widely prescribed. Too often, clinicians focused at the personality traits of *patients* to predict addiction instead of the addictive potential of the drugs themselves. Moreover, when using measures like long-term pain control, functionality and return to work, the benefits of opioids have not even been demonstrated. Even for short-term use, medications like OxyContin, Percocet and Vicodin and patches can pose significant concerns and can delay recovery. Moreover, cessation of the medication can cause significant withdrawal symptoms characterized by sweating, nausea, vomiting, and flu-like symptoms, seizures and, ironically, increased pain.

In a very limited number of closely monitored patients, opioids may allow patients to maintain work, social and recreational activities but when opioids are used inappropriately, quality of life clearly goes down. Patients become increasingly physically inactive, depressed, and fail to use other physical, psychological, and complementary therapies offered with multidisciplinary care. In these instances, opioids produce dependency on the healthcare system instead of self-responsibility in managing pain. It is very easy to tell which of your patients are motivated to try the different modalities found in multidisciplinary treatment and which are just seeking drugs. In light of opioids' limited use in long-term management, narrow safety profile, addiction potential and societal diversion, most pain medicine associations, and the US Food and Drug Administration have revised their guidelines in recent years.

References

AACVPR. (2015). *Cardiac rehabilitation fast facts*. Retrieved from https://www.aacvpr.org/about/aboutcardiacpulmonaryrehab/tabid/560/default.aspx

Airaksinen, O., Brox, J. I., Cedraschi, C., Hildebrandt, J., Klaber-Moffett, J., Kovacs, F., et al. (2006). European guidelines for the management of chronic nonspecific low back pain. *European Spine Journal, 15*(Suppl. 2), 192–300.

American College of Occupational and Environmental Medicine. (2007). Low back disorders. In K. T. Hegmann (Ed.), *Occupational medicine practice guidelines: Evaluation and manage-*

ment of common health problems and functional recovery in workers (2nd ed.). Elk Grove
Village, IL: ACOEM.
Brill, S. (2015). *America's bitter pill: Money, politics, back-room deals, and the fight to fix our broken healthcare system*. New York: Random House.
Chou, R., Atlas, S., Stanos, S., & Rosenquist, R. (2009a). Nonsurgical interventional therapies for low back pain. *Spine, 34*(10), 1078–1093.
Chou, R., Baisden, J., Caragee, E., Resnick, D., Shaffer, W., & Loeser, J. (2009b). Surgery for low back pain. *Spine, 34*(10), 1094–1109.
Chou, R., Loeser, J., Owens, D., Rosenquist, R., Atlas, S., Baisden, J., et al. (2009c). Interventional therapies, surgery, and interdisciplinary rehabilitation for low back pain. *Spine, 34*(10), 1066–1077.
Chou, R., Qaseem, A., Snow, V., Casey, D., Cross, J. T., Jr., Shekelle, P., et al. (2007). Diagnosis and treatment of low back pain: A joint clinical practice guideline from the American College of Physicians and the American Pain Society. *Annals of Internal Medicine, 147*(7), 478–491.
Chou, R., & Shekelle, P. (2010). Will this patient develop persistent disabling back pain? *Journal of the American Medical Association, 303*(13), 1295–1302.
Deyo, R., & Chou, R. (2014). Back pain. The evidence for nonsurgical management. In K. Burchiel (Ed.), *Surgical management of pain*. New York: Thieme.
Deyo, R., & Weinstein, J. (2001). Low back pain. *New England Journal of Medicine, 344*, 363–370.
Ditre, J. W., Zale, E. L., Koshiba, J. D., & Zvolensky, M. J. (2013). A pilot study of pain related anxiety and smoking dependence motives among persons with chronic pain. *Experimental and Clinical Psychopharmacology, 21*(6), 443–449.
Ekholm, O., Gronbaek, M., Peuckmann, V., & Sjogren, P. (2009). Alcohol and smoking behavior in chronic pain patients: The role of opioids. *European Journal of Pain, 13*(6), 606–612.
Frellick, M. (2014, June 30). One in five us adults use tobacco products. *Medscape Medical News*.
Frieden, J. (2011, March 28). AAPM: State of mind can turn acute pain to chronic. *MedPage Today*.
Groopman, J. (2007). *How doctors think* (pp. 167–181). New York: Houghton.
Hadler, N. (2009). *Stabbed in the back*. Chapel Hill: University of North Carolina Press.
Hadler, N., Tait, R., & Chibnall, J. (2007). Back pain in the work place. *Journal of the American Medical Association, 297*(14), 1594.
Haldeman, S., & Dagenais, S. (2008). A supermarket approach to the evidence-informed management of chronic low back pain. *The Spine Journal, 8*, 1–7.
Hanscom, D. (2012). *Back in control*. Seattle, WA: Vertus Press.
Haswell, K., Gilmour, J., & Moore, B. (2008). Clinical decision rules for identification of low back pain patients with neurologic involvement in primary care. *Spine, 33*(1), 68–73.
Hazards, R. (1994). Occupational low back pain. *American Pain Society Journal, 3*(2), 101–106.
In W. Fordyce (Ed.). (1995). *Back pain in the work place: Management of disability in nonspecific conditions*. Report of the task force on pain in the work place. Seattle, WA: International Association for the Study of Pain.
Interdisciplinary Program on Pain and Suffering, Flor, H., & Turk, D. (2011). *Pain: An integrated bio-behavioral approach*. Washington, DC: The International Association for the Study of Pain.
Kinkade, S. (2007). Evaluation and treatment of acute low back pain. *American Family Physician, 75*(8), 1181–1188.
MacDonald, D., Moseley, G. L., & Hodges, P. W. (2009). Why do some patients keep hurting their back? Evidence of ongoing back muscle dysfunction during remission from recurrent back pain. *Pain, 142*(3), 183–188.
Marcus, N. (2012). *End back pain forever*. New York: Atria Books.
McKenzie, R. (1980). *Treat your own back* (9th ed., pp. 5–9). Minneapolis, MN: Orthopedic Physical Therapy Products.
Mixter, W., & Barr, J. (1934). Rupture of the intervertebral disc with involvement of the spinal canal. *New England Journal of Medicine, 211*, 210–215.

National Institute of Neurological Disorders and Stroke. (2014). *Low back pain fact sheet.*

Nordqvist, C. (2013, May 9). Antibiotics may cure 40 % of chronic back pain cases. *Medical News Today.*

Patel, A. T., & Ogle, A. A. (2000). Diagnosis and management of acute low back pain. *American Family Physician, 61*(6), 1779–1786, 1789–1790.

Rasmussen, C., Nielsen, G., Hansen, V., Jensen, O., & Schioettz-Christensen, B. (2005). Rates of lumbar disc surgery before and after implementation of multidisciplinary nonsurgical spine clinic. *Spine, 30*(21), 2469–2473.

Rogers, J., Stout, C., Mack, B., Whitney, N., & Loughran, L. (2013). Return-to-work outcomes in non-operative lumbar cases following an evidence-based post-surgical rehabilitation program. *Disability Medicine, 9*(1), 3–9.

Sarno, J. (1984). *Mind over back pain: A radically new approach to the diagnosis and treatment of back pain.* New York: Berkley Books.

Shanti, B., & Shanti, I. (2014). Updates on smoking and low back pain. *Practical Pain Management, 14*(10), 23–26.

Spine-Health. (2014). *Quitting smoking before a spinal fusion.* Retrieved from http://www.spine-health.com/wellness/stop-smoking/quitting-smoking-a-spinal-fusion

Vranceanu, A., Barsky, A., & Ring, D. (2009). Psychosocial aspects of disabling musculoskeletal pain. *Journal of Bone and Joint Surgery, 91*(8), 2014–2018.

Weingarten, T. N., Podduturu, V. R., Hooten, W. M., Beebe, T. J., & Warner, D. O. (2008). An assessment of the association between smoking status, pain intensity, and functional interference in patients with chronic pain. *Pain Physician, 11*(5), 643–653.

Wheeler, A., et al. (2013, January 8). Low back pain and sciatica. *Medscape.*

Willems, P., Staal, J., Walenkamp, G., & de Bie, R. (2013). Spinal fusion for chronic low back pain. *Spine, 13*, 99–109.

Chapter 10
Other Common Pain Problems: Fibromyalgia, Myofascial Pain Syndrome and Complex Regional Pain Syndromes

In the previous chapter we addressed low back pain (LBP or back pain) which is responsible for the majority of visits to a physician by pain patients.

In this chapter, we will address complex regional pain syndrome (CRPS), fibromyalgia syndrome (FM), and myofascial pain syndrome (MPS) which are less common than LBP but are also challenging to understand and treat. Like all chapters in this book, the concepts are presented only as a broad overview of common chronic pain conditions and not a comprehensive discussion of the nuances of the conditions and their treatment. I recommend that you explore these topics further, as they relate to your practice, using the materials suggested in the references section of this book.

Pain Syndromes

Unlike a disease with a clear cause and treatment, syndromes like CRPS, fibromyalgia syndrome (FM) and MPS are a collection of symptoms that form a distinct pattern and suggest a certain condition. These are *not* diseases with a clear or consensus-based cause, a typical course and a set of specific treatments with resolution or control of the disease and associated symptoms. Bacterial pneumonia, meningitis, rheumatoid arthritis, and multiple sclerosis are clearly diseases in which the exact cause and treatment are known. It is ironic that when a disease and its treatment are well known, there are fewer books written about it than vague conditions and syndromes. There is certainly not an entire shelf at the bookstore about bacterial pneumonia as there is, for example, for low back pain or migraine!

A syndrome lacks clear laboratory, X-ray and other consistent clinical findings and its symptoms can be vague and do not all have to be present in a patient for a differential diagnosis, though a number of the symptoms do need to be present. For example depression is a syndrome which, in its mild forms, may be referred to as dysthymia which is Greek for "bad state of mind." While dysthymia may be characterized by a sad mood, eating and sleep disturbances, and other symptoms, when it

© Springer International Publishing Switzerland 2015
S. Vasudevan, *Multidisciplinary Management of Chronic Pain*,
DOI 10.1007/978-3-319-20322-5_10

becomes severe or long-lasting it is considered the syndrome of depression and may be treated by counseling and/or medication.

Pain syndromes are a difficult area of pain medicine because they are often judgment calls which benefit from clinicians' experience. For example, I have seen and treated CRPS for years so have little trouble recognizing what is and is not the condition. Those who see CRPS rarely will have more questions.

Both CRPS and FM are simultaneously over- and underdiagnosed in our current healthcare system. Twenty or more years ago, there was a lack of clinician awareness about the syndromes and patients were treated symptomatically with unimodal care instead of holistically with a multidisciplinary approach. While patients with both syndromes might have accompanying depression or anxiety or other psychological symptoms, the conditions are definitely not "in their mind." Anyone who has seen an edematous and discolored limb affected by CRPS, for example, does not doubt the condition's physical basis.

While better awareness of the conditions can be valuable, there is a downside. As reimbursement patterns shift and medications become more aggressively marketed, the syndromes can be overdiagnosed. We need to be careful with such diagnoses, especially when a patient is in the Workers' Compensation or other disability system in which there might be dueling parties and financial judgments at stake. We explored the requirements of many US disability systems in Chap. 7, Evaluation of Disability in Patients with Chronic Pain. We also must be careful to not needlessly alarm patients by giving them a serious diagnosis.

Another problem with diagnosing pain syndromes is that they can coexist and overlap with arthritic, rheumatic, autoimmune, inflammatory, and psychological conditions. For example, a patient may have MPS and fibromyalgia concurrently. A limb that exhibits temperature, color, and trophic changes may not be CRPS but *disuse* from not using a limb for other pain-related reasons. As with most chronic pain conditions, pain syndromes can be accompanied by anxiety, depression, disuse and self-neglect which can create additional symptoms.

Fibromyalgia and Myofascial Pain

When it comes to FM and MPS, there are two medical misconceptions which complicate diagnosis and treatment. The first is that they are the same condition which they are indubitably not, as you will see in Table 10.1. Dunteman calls the frequent confusion a "tragedy" since "myofascial pain may be effectively treated, while fibromyalgia 'cures' are unlikely" (Dunteman 2004).

The second misconception is that fibromyalgia is an "exclusion diagnosis" after other conditions are ruled out. While it is true that FM can mimic other conditions, and there are disagreements about criteria for a FM diagnosis and objective lab/diagnostic tests are lacking, a clinical diagnosis of fibromyalgia is possible as we will see in this chapter.

Table 10.1 Is it fibromyalgia or myofascial pain?

Fibromyalgia	Myofascial Pain
Central nervous system involvement with both peripheral and central sensitization	A peripheral localized muscle problem
Tender points diagnosis	Trigger point diagnosis
Widespread pain	Regional pain in specific muscles
11 of 18 tender points respond	Trigger points—taut palpable bands of muscles
Stiffness especially on wakening	ROM, posture, and pain
May or may not follow illness—usually no specific cause or association with injury	May follow injury but mostly spontaneous
Fatigue	Not usually linked to fatigue
Sleep problems	Not usually linked to sleep problems
Cognition/memory problems	Not linked to cognition/memory problems
Centralized "pain magnification"	Does not usually centralize
Treated with drugs and counseling	Treated with stretching/mechanics/education
Usually does not fully resolve/controllable	Usually resolves with time, education, and treatment
Female predominance, 7 to 1	Female predominance, 3 to 1

While the conditions have different etiologies, diagnostic methods and treatments—fibromyalgia is often categorized under the emerging umbrella terms "central sensitivity/sensory amplification syndromes" and myofascial pain is a local muscle problem—both are soft tissue pain syndromes. Notably, both are also well treated with multidisciplinary care.

Myofascial Pain Syndrome and Its Diagnosis

Myofascial pain is a musculoskeletal disorder that accounts for 85–93 % of pain clinic visits, 30 % of general medical visits, and 21 % of orthopedic visits (Chowdhury and Goldstein 2014). Clinically, MPS is characterized by aching or pain in the soft tissues—muscles, ligaments, and tendons—tightness, stiffness, and occasional neurological symptoms like tingling, numbness, or other strange sensations. It is caused by myofascial "trigger points." Patients may also complain about dizziness, swelling, and feelings of warmth or coldness in the affected areas, sometimes affected by weather.

MPS generally presents as *regional pain*, which may involve the trapezius, scalene, and sternocleidomastoid muscles and pelvic girdle. It is usually triggered after a muscle injury when it is referred to as posttraumatic MPS, though it can frequently occur without a precipitating event or develop gradually. Sometimes microtrauma, vitamin deficiencies, chronic stress, chronic infection, hypothyroidism, hypoglycemia, hypouricemia, radiculopathy, and depression can contribute to the development of MPS (Chowdhury and Goldstein 2014).

Table 10.2 Diagnostic criteria for myofascial pain syndrome

Trigger points	Elicits radiating pain when tight tender muscle is palpated
Local twitch responses (LTR)	Contractions of and around taut band
Regional pain	Remains localized in a muscle or region
Taut band in muscle	Exhibits tenderness, "ropey" consistency of muscle palpated
Trigger point treatments relieve pain	Injections, "spray and stretch," proper posture, conditioning exercises, PT, relieve or eliminate pain

When you examine a MPS patient, you will usually find muscles have become shortened and tight with a *palpable taut band* within the muscle belly, attributed to increased acetylcholine, ACh receptor activity, and/or changes in hydrolysis. Muscle hyperactivity is seen which, because it increases muscle demand, can lead to hypo-perfusion, ischemia, hypoxia, and a cascade of pain-producing neurovasoreactive substances (Chowdhury and Goldstein 2014). The hyperactive muscle(s) produces limited ROM, reduced function, disuse syndromes and, sometimes fatigue and difficulty with sleep.

While this chapter is not intended to provide a complete clinical guideline, MPS is diagnosed on the basis of an assessment of regional pain, taut muscles, trigger points, and positive twitch responses as shown in Table 10.2. Trigger points, when compressed, produce pain both locally and at referred locations; for example, a trigger point in the scalene muscles of the neck may produce pain in the hand when compressed. The unique distribution of pain in MPS trigger points assists the diagnosis. If a trigger point does not cause myotomal radiation it is not diagnostic for MPS or useful in MPS treatment.

Physiologically, Chowdhury and Goldstein suggest that MPS trigger points "contain areas of sensitized, low-threshold nociceptors (free nerve endings) with dysfunctional motor end plates" (2014). "These motor plates connect to an end group of sensitized sensory motor neurons in charge of transmitting pain information from the spinal cord to the brain." Not surprisingly, inactivation of trigger points is the primary treatment for MPS and will reduce pain. However, patients should be cautioned that overuse, overstretching, and psychological distress or anxiety can reactivate trigger points after they have healed.

There are many individuals who may continue to complain of pain after a muscle strain which is sometimes termed posttraumatic MPS. In the medicolegal context such as in work injuries and car accidents that may have initiated the muscle strain, the presence of pain and stiffness, with mild diffuse pain on touching, does *not* constitute posttraumatic MPS even though it is soft tissue pain. When physicians and healthcare providers label such patients as having posttraumatic MPS and provide ongoing physical or chiropractic therapy or medications and injection of tender areas (calling them "trigger point injections") they not only do a disservice to the patient, they add to the medical and legal and societal costs of health care. Clearly, MPS should not be a catch-all diagnosis.

I would label a patient as having MPS when he meets these criteria:

1. The pain is a muscle or regional muscle group
2. There is a palpable taut band of muscle (ropey consistency of muscle)
3. There is a trigger point characterized by a twitch response
4. Palpation of the trigger point leads to reproduction of the patient's pain and the pain radiates in a myotomal not nerve pattern
5. The trigger point can be inactivated with physical therapy (stretch, myofascial release, and injections)

A useful resource for helping you assess and treat trigger points is *Myofascial Pain and Dysfunction: The Trigger Point Manual Volumes 1 and 2* (Simons and Travell 1998).

Treating Myofascial Pain Syndrome

Both the treatment of myofascial pain syndrome and fibromyalgia start with reassurance — letting the patient know that he does not have a progressive or crippling disease. While MPS can rarely become or coexist with fibromyalgia, MPS of a specific muscle in a regional distribution is usually a time-limited condition with healing seen in between 2 and 12 weeks. MPS does not require or respond to surgery or require ongoing medication.

MPS can be treated invasively with injections of trigger points with a combination of local anesthetic and steroid. It can also be treated manually by dry needling, although there are no long-term evidence-based studies, despite the modality's theoretical rationale. These trigger point injections should be a mutual decision reached with the patient and always part of multimodal treatment that includes stretching, posture, relaxation, and empowerment through education, stressing self-efficacy. Patients should be educated to exercise after the acute phase and to recognize, accept, and incorporate their awareness of the difference between "hurt" (which implies pain) and "harm" (which implies damage/reinjury) in their rehabilitation.

Interestingly, this is how many athletic injuries are treated in sports medicine, including those of quarterbacks and other football players. The injured athlete is moved from injury to healing with a graded exercise program that gradually progresses to higher levels of activity. It is ironic that even though multidisciplinary care and physical therapy are the basis of sports medicine, our healthcare system is phasing them out in favor of unimodal treatment.

Manual methods and/or physical therapy should be used for patients presenting with new, acute trigger points or trigger points not easily accessible by injection such as psoas muscles (Chowdhury and Goldstein 2014). If you and the patient decide to employ injections, local anesthetics such as lidocaine are usually introduced into the trigger points, with or without cortisone. The very insertion of needles can sometimes modify pain sensations and some studies have found that needles with no medication at all — called dry needling — can be effective, though more research into its effectiveness is required.

Table 10.3 Treatments for myofascial pain syndrome

Trigger point injections	Lidocaine, cortisone; "dry needling"; part of multidisciplinary care
Physical/mechanical treatments	Heat, stretching, exercise, aerobic conditioning, rarely temporary TENS
Physical therapy	Address dysfunctional posture, weak muscles, increase muscle length and range of motion
"Spray and stretch"	Stretching with fluoromethane, ethyl chloride sprays (Stretch is action; spray is distraction) works well with localized pain
Medication	Anti-inflammatory, NSAIDs, sleep medication (for brief period only to increase function)
Psychological treatment	Cognitive Behavioral, relaxation therapy when chronic MPS exceeds 6 months
Education	Assurance: not progressive or crippling condition; "hurt" versus "harm" education
Self-efficacy	Commitment to home program and self-care; self-responsibility, avoiding dependence on medical, chiropractic and passive therapies

Dunteman cautions that injections should not be regarded as a "cure" but rather as an "adjunct" to help a patient address dysfunctional postures and movements (2004). Anti-inflammatory drugs can be useful for short periods of time but opioids are to be avoided as they are in most chronic pain conditions. While for a time, opioids were increasingly used in minor pain conditions in the United States, the pendulum has definitely swung back to avoiding opioids beyond the first 2–4 weeks, only to assist in increasing activity and function. The risks of dependence and addiction outweigh their use and, on a long-term basis, they are ineffective and may even worsen pain symptoms.

Dysfunctional postures such as a forwardly displaced shoulder girdle or forward rotation of the pelvis and abdominal muscle weakness and hip flexor tightness are frequently behind MPS. In my clinical experience, the most effective physical treatment for MPS is stretching followed by vigorous aerobic exercise and conditioning with a cool down period. The patient should commit to a regular home program of the above to keep functional levels and trigger points inactive. Common MPS treatments are seen in Table 10.3.

Because of its postural components, MPS is ideally treated with multidisciplinary care and especially responsive to physical therapy, myofascial release and educating patients about the condition so they are motivated to maintain a home program of exercise and stretching.

Fibromyalgia and Its Diagnosis

As we have noted, fibromyalgia is often confused with MPS. MPS and FM are separate conditions with different etiologies, treatments, and prognoses. Both, however, respond well to multidisciplinary care as opposed to uncoordinated, unimodal care (Masters 2014).

The first modern description of fibromyalgia emerged in 1972 when Hugh Smythe first described criteria for the diagnosis of "fibrositis" (a term coined by Gowers in early 1900s), which included the presence of widespread pain and tenderness at many of the points that were eventually incorporated in the 1990 American College of Rheumatology (ACR) criteria (Harden et al. 2014). The term fibromyalgia comes from the Latin word fibra for fibrous tissue and the Greek words myos and algos for muscle and pain respectively and was adopted in 1976 and eventually, as noted incorporated by the ACR in 1990.

Approximately five million adults in the United States have fibromyalgia syndrome which strikes patients at an average age of 30 and 50 years, The largest demographic for FM is women aged 55–64 report White et al. (Karvelas and Vasudevan 2011). Because of the lack of objective imagery or laboratory findings to confirm FM, it has erroneously been cast as a psychogenic disorder or even a result of industrialized culture. Russell, however, reports that FM is also seen in nonindustrialized countries. Certainly emotional and cognitive symptoms are part of the syndrome by they do not explain its pathogenesis.

Perhaps no chronic pain condition is so complicated or paradoxical in its diagnosis: A FM designation requires that other conditions be ruled out *but is not merely an exclusionary diagnosis*. A FM designation is based on the subjective and clinical findings but it is not *just a symptom-based diagnosis*.

It is not the purpose of this chapter to provide complete treatment guidelines for FM but a basic familiarity with this condition will help you better serve your patients. While widespread pain above and below the waist lasting for more than 3 months is the primary FM symptom, Table 10.4 shows the breadth of symptoms that may be present in a patient.

Table 10.4 Possible presenting symptoms of fibromyalgia

Widespread pain
Joint pain tenderness
Muscle tenderness
Fatigue
Morning stiffness
Anxiety
Paresthesia
Depression
Headache
Sleep disturbances
Feeling cold
Non restful sleep
Dry itchy eyes/blurred vision
Changes in bowel habits/abdominal pain, irritable bowel
Bladder symptoms
Jaw pain
Memory/cognitive problems ("fibro fog")
Rash, hives, sun sensitivity
Ringing in ears/hearing difficulty
Changes in appetite and food taste

Table 10.5 Tender points to consider in a fibromyalgia diagnosis

Occiput	Bilateral, at suboccipital muscle insertions
Low cervical	Bilateral, at anterior aspects of intertransverse spaces at C5–C7
Trapezius	Bilateral, at midpoint of upper border
Supraspinatus	Bilateral, at origins above scapula spine near medial border
Second rib	Bilateral, at second costochondral junctions just lateral to junctions on upper surfaces
Lateral epicondyle	Bilateral, 2 cm distal to epicondyles
Gluteal	Bilateral, in upper outer quadrants of buttocks in the anterior fold of muscle
Greater trochanter	Bilateral, posterior to trochanteric prominence
Knee	Bilateral, at medial fat pad proximal to joint line

In 1990, the ACR introduced criteria for a fibromyalgia diagnosis which were based on the presence of widespread pain and tenderness in 11 areas of 18 possible "tender points" as shown in Table 10.5.

Since the introduction of ACR criteria for fibromyalgia in 1990, there have been objections and calls for clarification. First, it was found that medical professionals rarely actually conducted tender point counts in clinical settings and that they sometimes did not know how, reducing the condition to a symptom-based diagnosis (Wolfe et al. 2010). Secondly, some felt the 1990 criteria overlooked the important cognitive and somatic symptoms that patients often report with FM like memory problems and fatigue. Thirdly, some medical professionals regard FM as a spectrum disorder and worried that a tender point orientation could preclude a spectrum diagnosis or incorrectly link fibromyalgia to peripheral muscle abnormality conditions.

There was even another problem: if a patient improved or his tender points decreased, he could fail to meet FM criteria yet still clearly have the condition.

In 2010, the ACR introduced new criteria acknowledging cognitive and affective symptoms and somatic symptoms like sleep problems, chest pain, fatigue, irritable bowel syndrome, bladder irritability, and headache (Russell 2011). Like the 1990 diagnostic criteria, the 2010 included a Widespread Pain Index and a Symptom Severity Scale for additional accuracy.

What Causes Fibromyalgia?

Like related pain syndromes, fibromyalgia is believed to be a disorder of increased central sensitization and decreased function of the descending pain inhibition systems (Clauw 2013). These disruptions, called descending inhibitory controls, which are part of decreased descending systems, result in abnormal temporal summation and sensory amplification (Karvelas and Vasudevan 2011). Even the perception of sound can be amplified in fibromyalgia patients reports Gary Jay, MD.

Fibromyalgia seems linked to genetic polymorphisms relating to serotoninergic, dopaminergic, and catecholaminergic systems but also no doubt has environmental factors which can include physical, sexual or emotional trauma, chronic stress or the aftermath of an acute illness. Abeles et al. state "fibromyalgia seems to be a final common pathway for a myriad of conditions, or combinations thereof, ranging from the psychosocial to the mechanical to the biological."

Abnormalities of the hypothalamic–pituitary–adrenal axis (HPA) have been described in patients with fibromyalgia and a number of studies show evidence of elevated cortisol levels, substance P, and decreased cortisol secretion in response to stress and corticotropin-releasing hormone stimulation. These changes may be an adaptive response of the body to chronic stress, rather than a biological abnormality specific to fibromyalgia syndrome.

Dunteman writes that FM patients show lower neurotransmitter levels, elevated substance P and their ACTH and norepinephrine releases in response to hyperglycemia are blunted in CSF assays. Sleep-induced prolactin and growth hormone release and heart rate response to exercise and vasoconstrictor response to acoustic and cold sensors are also blunted reports Dunteman (2004).

FM may involve an abnormality in the activation of N-methyl-D-aspartate (NMDA) receptors, linked to the condition's hyperalgesia suggests a clinical update from the International Association for the Study of Pain (IASP), noting that elevated nitric oxide plasma levels were seen following a vein distension test (2003). Proposing an "intriguing link between aberrant stress responses and… possible dysregulation of proinflammatory cytokines," the Association points out that fibromyalgia patients are more likely to develop hypotension during an orthostatic stressor.

Fibromyalgia patients demonstrate distinctive reactions to N-methyl-D-aspartate receptor (NMDAR) antagonist drugs like ketamine and buspirone and Wood and Holman suggest that dopamine-mediated actions explain a large part of fibromyalgia syndrome (2009). They term the role of DA in fibromyalgia "An Elephant Among Us."

Abnormalities of the HPA and other chemical/neurotransmitter disturbances are not unique to fibromyalgia but are also seen in stress-related disorders such as chronic fatigue syndrome, chronic pelvic pain, and posttraumatic stress disorder.

Fibromyalgia symptoms can also overlap with irritable bowel syndrome, multiple chemical sensitivities, tension and migraine headaches, interstitial cystitis, temporomandibular disorders, depression and anxiety and other inflammatory, endocrine and psychological disorders. Some clinicians regard the comorbid conditions as part of a fibromyalgia "spectrum."

A differential diagnosis for fibromyalgia syndrome should include rheumatoid arthritis, systemic lupus erythematosus, Lyme disease, hepatitis C, osteomalacia, polymyositis, Sjogren syndrome, polymyalgia rheumatica, myositis, myopathies, ankylosing spondylitis, hypothyroidism, and neuropathies. Clearly these conditions do not *exclude* fibromyalgia since there can be coexistence, but note that what appear to be fibromyalgia symptoms may indicate another disorder. Notably physical or emotional trauma and physical or sexual abuse can also be part of fibromyalgia patients' histories.

Treating Fibromyalgia

There may be no chronic pain condition that better demonstrates the benefits of a multidisciplinary treatment than fibromyalgia. Even clinicians who operate from a purely biomedical model of pain, concede that the baffling array of somatic, sensory, and cognitive symptoms fibromyalgia presents is best treated with multidisciplinary care, especially because a cornerstone of multidisciplinary care is patient education, encouragement, and empowerment—features that are often lacking in uncoordinated, unimodal care. Jay (2014), Argoff (2011), Dunteman (2004) and the International Association for the Study of Pain (2003) note the optimal treatment for FM is a multidisciplinary team with the participation of a physician, psychotherapist, nurse, physical and occupational therapists, and other allied health professionals as needed.

Yet, writes Jay with sardonic humor, when it comes to the proven benefits of multidisciplinary treatment—decreased pain, fatigue, depression, anxiety, improved quality of life and function, and decreased medical costs—insurers have obtuse "mural dyslexia": the inability to read the handwriting on the wall about better outcomes.

Like other chronic pain conditions, fibromyalgia is rarely cured but can be well managed through physical therapy, education, pharmacotherapy, psychological counseling, and other multidisciplinary care as seen in Table 10.6. Care often begins with reassuring patients and encouraging them in self-efficacy, self-management, and self-care.

Medications

As we discussed in Chap. 6, antidepressants and antiseizure medications are useful in chronic pain treatment because of their neuromodulatory effects. Other medications are also used in fibromyalgia as seen in Table 10.7.

Table 10.6 Fibromyalgia treatment—overview

Pharmacotherapy	Tricyclic antidepressants, antiseizure drugs, SNRIs and more
Physical modalities	Physical and occupational therapies
Psychological counseling	Cognitive Behavioral, relaxation therapy; self-efficacy/self-responsibility
Alternative and complementary	Acupuncture, massage, herbal/nutritional supplements
Exercise	Strength and aerobic training

Table 10.7 Medications used in fibromyalgia

Tricyclic antidepressants	Amitriptyline, imipramine, clomipramine, nortriptyline, desipramine and maprotiline
Selective norepinephrine reuptake inhibitors (SNRI)	Venlafaxine, duloxetine, milnacipran levomilnacipran
Antiseizure drugs	Gabapentin, pregabalin
Analgesics	Tramadol is only useful opioid
Anti-inflammatory drugs	NSAIDs, steroids not useful; cyclobenzaprine may be useful
Other	Lidocaine, anesthetics, possibly growth hormones and substrate drugs

Tricyclic Antidepressants

Before SSRI and SNRI antidepressants, depression was often treated with tricyclic antidepressants like amitriptyline, imipramine, clomipramine, nortriptyline, desipramine, and maprotiline. As the drugs were replaced as first-line antidepressants, they were recruited as useful agents in dampening pain in some chronic pain conditions. Amitriptyline is probably the most well-studied tricyclic antidepressant used for the treatment of fibromyalgia, but others are used and have been studied.

While tricyclic antidepressants clearly inhibit the reuptake of serotonin and norepinephrine, the exact mechanism of their action on fibromyalgia and other neuropathic pain remains unknown. It is likely, though, that their action upon pain is separate and distinct from their action on depression pain relief since it is achieved at lower doses and in much shorter time intervals than their effects as antidepressants. Tricyclic antidepressants are especially useful in treating sleep problems in FM patients but their anticholinergic, antiadrenergic, antihistaminergic, and quinidine-like side effects can limit their use, especially in the elderly. They are not specifically FDA approved for FM.

Selective Norepinephrine Reuptake Inhibitors

Selective Norepinephrine Reuptake Inhibitor (SNRIs) like venlafaxine (Effexor), duloxetine (Cymbalta), milnacipran (Savella), and levomilnacipran (Fetzima) are also used in FM. A Cochrane review of three double-blind randomized controlled trials investigating the use of duloxetine (Cymbalta) for treatment of fibromyalgia syndrome found that a daily dose of 60 mg reduced pain by 50 % though a lower dose was ineffective (Karvelas and Vasudevan 2011). Duloxetine is FDA-approved for fibromyalgia syndrome. Common side effects are dizziness, dry mouth, headache, and constipation.

Venlafaxine (Effexor), another SNRI, produced significant improvement in pain in an open-label pilot study yet showed no pain improvement in a randomized, placebo-controlled, double-blind trial at a lower dose. It is possible that these conflicting results reflect a lack of inhibition of norepinephrine reuptake at a lower dose. Venlafaxine is not FDA approved for FM.

Milnacipran, another drug the FDA has approved for FM is thought to mildly inhibit NMDA receptors in addition to blocking the reuptake of NE and 5HT. Two large double-blind randomized controlled trials showed evidence for pain reduction in the treatment of fibromyalgia syndrome—the first registering more than 30 % reduction in pain—and both trials improved global well-being and physical function. Side effects with milnacipran included constipation, nausea, sweating, hot flushes, dry mouth, and hypertension.

Antiseizure Drugs

Antiseizure drugs are often used for the treatment of fibromyalgia syndrome and include gabapentin (Neurontin) and pregabalin (Lyrica). While the exact mechanism of action of these drugs remains unknown, it probably relates to the drugs' ligands binding to voltage-gated calcium channels and modulating calcium ion influx. This binding likely stabilizes hyperexcited neurons, inhibiting the release of excitatory neurotransmitters such as glutamate and substance P, which are believed to be involved in pain processing.

Pregabalin has been approved by the FDA for the treatment of fibromyalgia syndrome since 2007. A Cochrane review of four double-blind randomized controlled trials found pregabalin efficacious for pain relief, including patient reports of improvement. The greatest response was seen at 225 mg twice daily and reported side effects included peripheral edema and weight gain.

Unlike pregabalin, gabapentin has not been approved by the FDA for the treatment of fibromyalgia but is often substituted for pregabalin because it is cheaper, though also less potent and, so, used at a higher dose. In a 12-week, randomized, double-blind, placebo-controlled trial, gabapentin was found to significantly improve pain and sleep though it did not significantly improve the mean tender point pain threshold or ratings of depression.

Analgesics

We have noted in many chapters in this book that chronic pain should seldom be treated with opioids which are linked to addiction and misuse and may actually be associated with an increased sensitivity to pain, referred to as opioid-induced hyperalgesia. In FM, opioids have reduced efficacy which may have a physiological cause: when challenged with the μ-opioid receptor PET, FM patients display reduced μ-opioid receptor binding potential within several regions of the brain, areas that modulate pain.

Despite several evidence-based guidelines that recommend SNRI and tricyclic antidepressants, antiseizure drugs and rarely tramadol, but not opioids, the latter remain the most commonly prescribed agents for this population. In fact, Masters reports that opioids account for 59 % of prescriptions given to the fibromyalgia population (2–14).

On the basis of my own decades of practice, I strongly believe cessation of opioids is the first step in beginning to treat chronic pain conditions, specifically fibromyalgia.

Tramadol, a weak opioid, may represent an exception to the cautions issued about opioid drugs. It has shown effectiveness in fibromyalgia both alone and in combination with acetaminophen. In a multicenter, double-blind, randomized, placebo-controlled study patients in the treatment group showed a greater than 50 % reduction in pain as well as an improvement in physical function with a combination of tramadol and acetaminophen.

Like other opioids, tramadol is a "clean" drug that is not associated with organ damage like NSAIDs. However, unlike other opioids, it does not produce the "high" which is behind the addiction and abuse potential of this drug class and I use it with select patients. As part of multidisciplinary treatment, tramadol is useful in helping patients improve their functioning by participating in therapies. More FM trials using tramadol alone would be helpful.

Anti-inflammatory Drugs

Although they are commonly used, there is no evidence that NSAIDs are useful in the treatment of fibromyalgia syndrome. Rossy et al. found that NSAIDs were not significantly associated with improvement in any outcome measure, though some studies have documented a "minor" benefit of ibuprofen when combined with the tricyclic antidepressant amitriptyline and naproxen when combined with cyclobenzaprine, a muscle relaxer (2011). Cyclobenzaprine, which has a chemical structure similar to tricyclics, is not approved for the treatment of FM but in some studies helped with sleep problems compared to placebo.

Similarly, there is no evidence for the benefit of steroids, which are potent anti-inflammatory drugs in the treatment of fibromyalgia syndrome and in one double-blind, placebo-controlled, crossover trial study evaluating the corticosteroid prednisone, a "trend towards deterioration" was actually reported.

Other Drugs

Okifuji and Turk note that other drugs have been tried in FM with varying results. Benzodiazepines and hypnotic drugs like zolpidem produced "little benefit for mood or sleep"; S-adenosylmethionine and 5-hydroxytryptophan showed "mixed success" and daily growth hormone improved hyperalgesia and perceived disability but "the high cost of such treatment limits its utility," write the researchers (2003). SP receptor agonists have not proved effective in human trials of FM patients despite their clear aberrations of Substance P levels writes Jay (2014). Malic acid, magnesium, and long-chain polyunsaturated fatty acids such as found in fish oil or lecithin have demonstrated some efficacy says Dunteman (2004).

Physical Treatments and Exercise

Exercise, whether aerobic or for strength and flexibility, correlates well with improved pain and function and global well-being in patients with fibromyalgia (Karvelas and Vasudevan 2011). However, many patients find it difficult to adhere to an exercise program and can benefit from encouragement and education. Also, an exercise program should be instituted slowly, aiming for a moderate level of intensity in order to avoid exacerbations of pain and encourage compliance.

A Cochrane review of exercise in fibromyalgia found that 12 weeks of moderate intensity aerobic training may improve well-being and physical function though not necessarily produce a reduction in pain or tender points. Strength training for 12 weeks, on the other hand, seemed to be correlated with large reductions in pain, tender points as well as improvements in global well-being and relief of depression though not a difference in physical function. Clearly, a combination of strength and moderate intensity aerobic training can be helpful in patients with fibromyalgia.

Psychological Treatment

Psychological factors affect pain in all chronic pain conditions and they are especially influential with fibromyalgia. Nielson et al. found, for example, FM patients who had an increased sense of control over pain, a conviction that they were not necessarily disabled by fibromyalgia and a clear distinction between "hurt" and "harm" experienced more positive outcomes. Cognitive Behavioral therapy, addressed in Chap. 4, improved coping with pain and reduced depressed mood and healthcare-seeking behavior in FM patients reported Bernardy et al. though actual reductions in pain or fatigue and improvement in sleep quality were not noted. Glombiewski et al. found similar results. As we saw in Chap. 4, Cognitive Behavioral and other therapies help in reducing illness conviction and depression and improving coping mechanisms. In addition to Cognitive Behavioral therapy, relaxation therapy, biofeedback, and mindfulness-based treatment have proved useful.

As we see in most chronic pain conditions, the best FM treatment uses a multidisciplinary approach, treating the "person" and not the "pain." It facilitates education about the condition and family participation, reduces illness behavior and encourages patients in self-efficacy and self-management. "The patient should be redirected from a sick role focus to a functional role, thereby helping the patient with self-respect, family, and social activity as well as possible employment," writes Dunteman (2004).

Complex Regional Pain Syndrome

CRPS dates back more than 100 years when it was described during the Civil War by Silas Weir Mitchell, MD, who treated soldiers' gunshot wounds and coined the term "causalgia," Greek for "burning pain." The swelling of the limbs/joints seen with causalgia was distinct from swelling from the wound itself, wrote Dr. Mitchell and seemed to stem from nerve injury, though it might be masked by the injury for a time. "Once fully established, it keeps the joint stiff and sore for weeks or months. When the acute stage has departed, the tissues become hard and partial ankylosis results," Dr. Mitchell wrote.

As the era of modern medicine began and rheumatologists and orthopedic surgeons started to see fractures, swollen wrists and shoulders with limited ranges of motion which bore causalgia-like symptoms, the terms "shoulder-hand syndrome" and "Sudeck's atrophy" began to be employed. By the 1950s, however, the condition began to be viewed as a syndrome involving the sympathetic nervous system, dystrophy and other symptoms and not necessarily caused by nerve injury. The term Reflex Sympathetic Dystrophy or RSD was born.

Since the 1990s, the term again has evolved and is now called CRPS on the basis of clearly defined features seen in Table 10.8.

In this section we will explore the many complications of CRPS which may have even deeper historical roots than the Civil War: Gierthmuhlen et al. note that CRPS displays the five cardinal signs of inflammation described by Celsus and Galen *2000 years ago*: dolor (pain), calor heat, rubor (redness), tumor (swelling), and functio laesa (loss of function) (2014).

Table 10.8 Key aspects of complex regional pain syndrome

Complex	Symptoms varied and dynamic between patients and within patient
Signs	Autonomic, cutaneous, vascular, motor or dystrophic changes and neuropathic
Regional	Symptoms spread to other regions, usually distal only—may move proximally from fingers, hand and to forearm; from feet to lower leg; does not typically start in the large joints of hips, knees, and shoulders or spine
Pain	Disproportionate to event; can be spontaneous and burning in quality; allodynia, dysesthesia, and hyperpathia
Syndrome	Constellation of events sufficient for a pattern to suggest the diagnosis
Treatment	Medical, physical, psychological, social, vocational factors must be addressed—multidisciplinary treatment best in subacute (6–12 weeks) and chronic (after 12 weeks)

Table 10.9 Presenting symptoms of CRPS

Allodynia
Hyperpathia
Dysesthesia
Edema
Trophic changes
Atrophy
Contracture
Increased sweating
Skin temperature changes
Patchy juxta-articular osteoporosis on X-rays and triphasic bone scan

Patients with CRPS will most frequently report burning pain followed by constant or occasional stabbing and shooting pain and/or deep aching. 86.9 % of patients presenting with CRPS have vasomotor abnormalities and 52.9 % have sudomotor changes including hyper/hypohidrosis (Indian Journal of Rheumatology 2014). Kinesophobia and motor weakness are also possible. Patients also may report muscle spasm and the "shakes," decreased range of motion and loss of strength or function.

CRPSs can be caused by sprains, fractures, crash injuries, blunt trauma and repetitive/cumulative trauma, surgery, M.I., stroke, and amputations but can also occur from unknown reasons. Gierthmuhlen et al. have noted that neglect phenomenon such as abnormal postures and contracture and mental health problems may also be linked to the condition (2014). Common presenting symptoms are seen in Table 10.9.

Diagnosing CRPS

A diagnosis of CRPS is not always easy. While some clinicians are still fairly unaware of the condition, *others may be overly focused and overdiagnose CRPS, when they cannot explain symptoms, even though many features of the syndrome are not identifiable.* Thus pain lasting beyond the healing period with swelling can be inappropriately attributed to CRPS even though the observed symptoms can come from disuse and "anticipatory fear," especially in medicolegal situations like work injuries and auto accidents. Clearly this leads to an unfortunate odyssey of treatment that includes a plethora of medications, nerve blocks, rest and inactivity, spinal cord stimulation, opioid prescriptions which increases the patient's illness and disability "convictions" and increases healthcare costs for everyone. *It is very important to not to let unexplained symptoms cause CRPS to be a "catch-all" diagnosis, especially because of the dangers of patients developing the conviction that they have a "chronic disease" which can become a self-fulfilling prophesy.*

Table 10.10 Categories required for CRPS diagnosis

One or more of these categories must be involved	
Sensory	Hyperalgesia/allodynia/dysesthesia/hyperpathia
Vasomotor	Asymmetrical swelling, temperature and color
Sudomotor/edema	Sweating, altered-usually increased
Motor	Decreased ROM, tremor
Trophic	Excessive growth, friability and thinning of nails, hair, skin on affected side
Injury/trauma	Spread of reactions beyond site of initial injury, distal to proximal; other side symptoms very rare

Table 10.11 Clinical presentations required for Budapest CRPS criteria

Sensory	Evidence of hyperalgesia (to pinprick) and/or allodynia (to light touch and/or deep somatic pressure and/or joint movement)
Vasomotor	Evidence of temperature asymmetry and/or skin color changes and/or asymmetry
Sudomotor/edema	Evidence of edema and/or sweating changes and/or sweating asymmetry
Motor/trophic	Evidence of decreased range of motion and/or motor dysfunction (weakness, tremor, dystonia) and/or trophic changes (hair, nail, skin)

Moreover, CRPS may be diagnosed on the basis of different criteria depending on the medical professional. A surgeon will suspect CRPS when there is excessive pain after surgery; an anesthesiologist will likely focus on excessive pain and complaints of cold and swelling in the affected area; a neurologist may look for neuropathic findings like allodynia, dysesthesia, and coldness and a rheumatologist will look for a positive bone scan and swelling.

It is widely agreed that a diagnosis of CRPS requires sensory, vasomotor symptoms (swelling, discoloration, temperature changes—mostly coldness), sudomotor symptoms (altered, usually increased sweating) and motor systems (muscle stiffness, decreased range of motion and strength and tremors) as shown in Table 10.10. *Asymmetrical differences in color, temperature, diffuse edema and pain and limited ROM are required for a CRPS diagnosis but other signs may or may not be present as we see in Tables* 10.10 *and* 10.11. Over half of CRPS cases do *not* respond to sympathetic blocks though lack of a positive response does not necessarily mean a condition is not CRPS.

Historically, CRPS has been diagnosed on the basis of the 1993 IASP criteria. But since their development, some pain experts have worried that, though the criteria accurately identify most cases of CRPS, they also tend to falsely identify neuropathic pain conditions that are not CRPS, potentially contributing to overdiagnosis and either inappropriate or unnecessary treatments. In 2004, a group of pain specialists meeting in Budapest developed what came to be called the "Budapest Criteria" for CRPS (Harden et al. 2010). The Budapest Criteria sought to correct

Table 10.12 Criteria to precede a CRPS diagnosis (my personal approach)

Asymmetrical differences in color, temperature, edema/swelling, sweating, pain; limited ROM, and other trophic changes of skin, hair, and nail growth	*Necessary*
Sensory, vasomotor, sudomotor-edema, and/or motor-trophic symptoms	*Necessary*
Occurrence or increase of above symptoms after use of the limb	*Possible*
Presence of symptoms in area larger than injury, usually distal to injury	*Possible*
Positive response to sympathetic block	*Possible*
Positive response to sudomotor function tests	*Possible*

nonempirical patient "self-reporting" by requiring that evidence of at least one sign in two or more of categories be apparent at the time of evaluation, as shown in Table 10.11.

Have advanced a "severity score" for CRPS for clinical decision making which includes intensity of pain, distress, functional impairments and bilateral asymmetries (2010). The researchers also found depression and anxiety prior to surgery could be predictors of CRPS. Levine and Saperstein identify small fiber neuropathy in RSD/CRPS though current electromyogram (EMG) is not useful in its detection, they write (2012).

While the differential diagnosis of CRPS can still be challenging, it is helpful to know which symptoms *must* be present and which *might* be present as shown in Table 10.12.

What Causes CRPS?

At the physiologic level, CRPS is theorized to occur from peripheral trauma which causes a circle of excitatory influence of postganglionic sympathetic axons on primary afferent fibers. The trauma or initiating event likely sparks chronic stimulation of visceral or deep somatic afferents producing sympathetically maintained pain (Gierthmuhlen et al. 2014). Neuropeptides and artificial synapses called "ephapses" are likely involved in increased sensitization in the dorsal horn.

Gierthmuhlen et al. write that the release of cytokines leads to peripheral sensitization and sympatho-afferent coupling which then causes central sensitization and maladaptive neuroplasticity resulting in central motor symptoms (2014). The cascade, write the researchers, can be exacerbated by catecholamines released by psychogenic stress.

Henry et al. also cite plasticity associated with pain states like CRPS, reporting that neuroimaging reveals abnormalities with the pain "matrix"—a group of cortical and subcortical brain regions, some of which are reversible (2011). Imaging shows decreased pain activation in brain regions when a subject is distracted and increased pain activation when the subject focuses on the pain, the researchers add. The idea of the pain matrix stems from Melzack and Wall's Gate Theory which we explored in Chap. 3. After changes in the pain matrix from an injury, the "gate" does not close and allows C-fibers, A-delta fibers and other chemical messengers to centralize.

Studies also demonstrate that chronic pain activates brain regions involved with cognitive and emotional pain processing in a way acute pain does not (Henry et al. 2011). Even memories of pain may alter a patient's "somatotopic map," say the researchers and can date back to the neonatal period. However, early pain experiences and memories *do* respond to psychological counseling and condition, the researchers add—again demonstrating the value of multidisciplinary treatment in chronic pain condition.

Another pain theory we reviewed in Chap. 3, the Mismatch Theory, may contribute to CRPS. Gierthmuhlen et al. observe that a mismatch between the "perceived location of a stimulus… and visuospatial frame of reference" could reduce pain in studied patients with chronic pain—an occurrence called visually induced analgesia. The phenomenon is especially relevant to CRPS patients, say the researchers, because "vision, body perception disturbance and pain perception are known to be closely linked" (2014). Specifically, CRPS patients who used prismatic goggles that produced a visual displacement toward the unaffected side, experienced a reduction in pain. Mirror therapy has also been used with CRPS patients write Gierthmuhlen et al.

More About CRPS

There are three stages of CRPS, depicted in Table 10.13. Pain, stiffness of joints and disability increase as the condition develops and some symptoms become irreversible so it is advisable to treat CRPS early—as soon as you make the differential diagnosis.

CRPS is frequently divided into two types of as we see in Table 10.14. CRPS I corresponds to RSD, symptoms not necessarily linked to a nerve injury. CRPS II corresponds to the causalgia Dr. Mitchell described during the Civil War and usually results from injury to large nerves such as the sciatic median or nerve. Symptoms appear more readily with CRPS II but it is more rarely seen by most practitioners than CRPS I.

Table 10.13 Stages of CRPS

Stage I—Mild	Symptoms soon after event; burning pain, edema, vasomotor/sudomotor changes, patchy osteoporosis on X-ray
Stage II—Moderate (after weeks/months)	Pain, edema spread; trophic changes; cold, pale, moist skin; muscle atrophy, osteoporosis, increased uptake on scan
Stage III—Severe	Severe tropic changes, allodynia, dysesthesia spread including to contralateral limb, throbbing pain, myoclonic movements, irreversible muscle atrophy, poor response to treatment

Table 10.14 The difference between CRPS I and CRPS II

CRPS 1	CRPS 11
Formerly reflex sympathetic dystrophy	Formerly causalgia
Initial injury mild without nerve injury	Partial injury to known large nerves or its major branches
Onset often takes a month	Onset often occurs immediately
Pain, disproportionate to inciting event	Pain disproportionate to inciting event
Edema, changes in skin blood flow, sudomotor activity at start of injury	Edema, changes in skin blood flow, sudomotor activity at any time
Pain not limited to area of injury	Pain not limited to the area of injury
No other conditions explaining pain and other findings	*No other conditions explaining pain and other findings*

Table 10.15 The "Mix" of treatment modalities for CRPS

Pharmacotherapy—typically tricyclic and SNRI antidepressants, antiseizure drugs; topical local anesthetics
Interventional approaches—blocks, spinal cord stimulation
Multidisciplinary rehabilitation-PT, OT, vocational, nursing/social worker
Psychological/psychiatric treatment, Cognitive Behavioral therapy, Reframing
Rarely surgery (except for SCS or "pump" in select patients; surgery is known to make CRPS worse)
Education/empowerment of the patient and family
All of the above in correct balance

Treating Complex Regional Pain Syndrome

CRPS is a multifaceted condition that requires multifaceted treatment and a multidisciplinary team. It is no coincidence that the IASP was founded by the anesthesiologist John Bonica, MD to use multidisciplinary treatment to address such pain conditions.

As an especially confounding pain condition, CRPS should be treated with a team that has input from a physician, physical therapist, occupational therapist, anesthesiologist, neurologist, physiatrist, neurosurgeon, psychiatrist/psychologist, rehabilitation nurse, and recreational/vocational therapists. All these disciplines blend together to form the right "mix" to adequately treat CRPS as seen in Table 10.15. In fact, the only drawback with a multidisciplinary program is, as Gierthmuhlen et al. have pointed out, we usually can't point to which modality "worked." The mix of treatments "makes investigation of a single mechanism-based treatment option difficult," they write (2014).

Because CRPS is characterized by peripheral, central, and pathophysiologic processes manifesting as motor weakness, dystonia, tremor, kinesiophobia and neglect, physical and occupational therapies and allied health disciplines are especially skilled at decreasing patients' kinesiophobia, edema, and stress loading of extremities.

Table 10.16 CRPS treatments provided by multidisciplinary rehabilitation

Physical therapist	Heat/cold, contrast baths, pressure loading, and proprioceptive training, TENS
Occupational therapist	Edema control (taping), massage compression garments, protective and functional orthotics
Health psychologist	Cognitive Behavior, relaxation, biofeedback therapy. Addresses depression, anxiety, fear avoidance. Reframing
Social worker/nurse	Involves family, support systems to help patient regain self-efficacy and activities
Vocational therapists	Coordinate return to work with employers and disability system representatives
Medication	Antidepressants, antiseizure drugs, NSAIDs, discourage opioids, benzodiazepines, and drugs of abuse
Surgical	Spinal stimulator, epidurals, IDDS (implanted morphine pumps); rarely dorsal root entry zone (DREZ) lesions and sympathectomy (not used currently or evidence-based)

In my own experience, a coordinated, integrated team can prevent and reverse disability in patients with CRPS using physical rehabilitation, psychological support and interventional/anesthesiology, pharmacotherapy and surgery as needed, especially when treatment is begun soon enough as seen in Table 10.15. *Multidisciplinary clinicians help patients desensitize their pain, increase their activities of daily living (ADLs) and progress towards their short and long-term goals through empathizing with but not reinforcing "pain behaviors"* as seen in Tables 10.15 and 10.16.

Using Cognitive Behavioral and relaxation therapies, CRPS patients receive education about the biopsychosocial factors behind their pain and principles which are usually lacking in unimodal care. They learn the difference between "hurt" (pain) and "harm" (damage), which helps them maintain their activities. In Chap. 8, we look at ways you can create your own multidisciplinary team.

Physical and Occupational Therapy

Physical therapists, for example, teach desensitization/stress loading, pacing, posture/ weight bearing, exercises and flexibility training, and proprioceptive neuromuscular facilitation/coordination. They can offer CRPS patients heat, electrical stimulation and TENS units to decrease pain as well as massage and exercises.

An especially effective maneuver for CRPS is "scrubbing"—a therapy discovered when a clinician noticed patients who worked as cleaners enjoyed faster recoveries from CRPS. Scrubbing involves moving an affected extremity in a back-and-forth motion while bearing weight on the limb. Physical and occupation therapists can also instruct patients in proper carrying with progressively heavy objects and correct walking with increased weight shifting employing balance-with-cues. OTs can outfit

Table 10.17 Useful treatments in CRPS

Level of treatment	Drugs	Physical modality/function
Peripheral	Lidocaine patches, NSAIDs, capsaicin, methyl salicylates, menthol, dexamethasone, arnica, sodium channel blockers, steroids, antiseizure drugs	Massage, electrical stimulation, stress loading cause desensitization, reduce edema, movement, functional exercises
Central/spine	SNRIs, gabapentin, pregabalin, TENS, stress loading	Dampen prostaglandin, substance P, aldolase, glutamate, and other neurotransmitters to quiet overactive nerves
Brain	SNRI, SSRIs, tricyclic antidepressants NOT opioids	Exercise, education, Cognitive Behavioral and relaxation techniques, therapy

patients with edema control-taping, massage compression garments, and protective and functional orthotics such as night splints.

For stress loading, a device called the Dystrophile has been useful. To relieve pain and stiffness while increasing blood circulation, fluidotherapy treatment is beneficial, especially because it is a dry heat which does not interfere with wound healing.

Medications

Because CRPS is mediated at three physiologic levels, pharmacotherapy also targets three distinct levels as shown in Table 10.17.

As we saw in Chap. 6, there are useful treatments for peripheral pain including those applied topically. In one study lidocaine, administered intravenously, reduced thermal and allodynic (Gierthmuhlen et al. 2014). Studies have not confirmed the efficacy of NSAIDs, carbamazepine, and sodium channel-modulating antiseizure drugs in CRPS (Gierthmuhlen et al. 2014). Oral steroids can be useful in patients with edema, raised temperature, and reddening though their effect on pain itself is not clear.

Many of the medications discussed in Chap. 6 such as tricyclic and SNRI antidepressants and antiseizure drugs like gabapentin and pregabalin are very useful in CRPS. Trials with medications, such as ketamine, TNF-blockers, bisphosphonates, and DSM have not revealed encouraging results (Gierthmuhlen et al. 2014).

Other Treatments

We have talked in previous chapters about the limitations of intervention medicine in some chronic pain conditions. However, when treating CRPS, sympathetic blocks, continuous peripheral blocks, epidural blocks, diagnostic, and therapeutic blocks can sometimes be useful and also used diagnostically. Similarly, while spinal cord

Table 10.18 Main points of this chapter	Pain syndromes are challenging to diagnose and treat
	Myofascial pain syndrome and fibromyalgia can coexist but have different causes and treatments
	Medications are helpful in FM and CRPS
	Multidisciplinary is the best treatment for MPS, FM, and CRPS
	Psychological counseling helps with coping and self efficacy

stimulation has limitations in chronic pain, CRPS is a condition in which it can be useful. As we noted in Chap. 3, Pain Theories and Factors Behind Chronic Pain and Chap. 6, Treating the Chronic Pain Patient, outcomes depend on careful patient selection.

In previous chapters we have looked at how "fear avoidance" and "learned disuse" can perpetuate pain or prevent recovery in chronic pain patients. In CRPS patients, "learned disuse" can maintain the CRPS condition by eliminating the normal tactile and proprioceptive input from the affected area that is necessary to restore normal central signal processing.

When edema and reduced circulation due to vasoconstriction are present as they often are in CRPS, learned disuse impairs the natural pumping action associated with movement that helps reduce local levels of catecholamines and metabolic byproducts. The result is that these chemical messengers build up in the patient, producing more pain and learned disuse which becomes a repeated cycle.

Pawl observes that many patients diagnosed with CRPS have "highly conditioned pain behaviors out of proportion to medical findings" and notes that as early as 1959, patients with what was still called Sudek's syndrome were seen to be "introspective and apprehensive" (Pawl 2000). Indeed, patients seeming to have CRPS have turned out to have factitious edema, writes Pawl—symptoms caused by self-inflicted tourniquets, irritations or blows to the arm. I have personally seen such factitious disorders in patients suspected of having CRPS.

As we prepare to look at the stories of patients with chronic pain who have recovered with multidisciplinary care in Chap. 11, let us review what we have learned in this chapter, seen in Table 10.18.

References

Argoff, C. (2011). Fibromyalgia: overview of etiology, pathophysiology, treatment, and management. *Pain Medicine News—Special Edition 9*(12), 74–78.

Chowdhury, N., & Goldstein, L. (2014). Diagnosis and management of myofascial pain syndrome. *Practical Pain Management, 12*, 2.

Clauw, D. (2013, December). What fibromyalgia teaches u about chronic pain. *Pain Medicine News—Special Edition.*

Mutagi, H., Guru, R., & Kapur, S. (2014). Complex regional pain syndrome (CRPS)—A brief review. *Indian Journal of Rheumatology, 9*(2), S26–S32.

Dunteman, E. D. (2004, July/August). Fibromyalgia and myofascial pain syndromes. *Pain Management*, pp. 26–29.

Gierthmuhlen, J., Binder, A., & Baron, R. (2014). Mechanism-based treatment in chronic regional pain syndromes. *Nature Reviews Neurology, 10*, 518–528.

Harden, R. N., et al. (2014). Development of a severity score for CRPS. *Pain, 151*(3), 870–876.

Henry, D. E., Chlodo, A. E., & Yang, W. (2011). Central nervous system reorganization in a variety of chronic pain states: A review. *PM R, 3*(12), 1116–1125.

International Association for the Study of Pain. (2003). Fibromyalgia syndrome: Prevalent and perplexing. *Pain Clinical Update, 11*(3), 2.

Jay, G. (2014a). Fibromyalgia: What clinicians need to know. *Practical Pain Management, 14*(7), 40.

Jay, G. (2014b). Fibromyalgia: What clinicians need to know. *Practical Pain Management, 14*(7), 45.

Karvelas, D., & Vasudevan, S. (2011). Fibromyalgia syndrome. *Pain Manag, 1*(6), 557–570.

Levine, T., & Saperstein, D. (2012, March). Reflex sympathetic dystrophy/complex regional pain syndrome and small fiber neuropathy. *Pain Medicine News*.

Masters, E. (2014, November/December). Are opioids being overprescribed for fibromyalgia? *Practical Pain Management*, pp. 19–20.

Okifuji, A., & Turk, D. (2003). Fibromyalgia syndrome: prevalent and perplexing. *Pain: Clinical Updates, 11*(3), 3. International Association for the Study of Pain (IASP).

Pawl, R. (2000). Controversies surrounding reflex sympathetic dystrophy: A review article. *Current Review of Pain, 4*(4), 259–267.

Russell, J. (2011, September). Fibromyalgia: Practical approaches to diagnosis and treatment. *Practical Pain Management*.

Simons, D. G., & Travell, J. G. (1998). *Myofascial pain and dysfunction: The trigger point manual* (Vol. 1, 2). Baltimore, MD: Williams & Wilkins.

Wolfe, F., Clauw, D., Fitzcharles, M., Goldenberg, D., Katz, R., Mease, P., et al. (2010). The American College of Rheumatology preliminary diagnostic criteria for fibromyalgia and measurement of symptom severity. *Arthritis Care & Research, 62*(5), 600–610.

Wood, P., & Holman, A. (2009). An elephant among us: The role of dopamine in the pathophysiology of fibromyalgia. *Journal of Rheumatology, 36*(2), 221–224.

Chapter 11
Patient Stories

Here are some stories about patients I have treated over the years. Many of these stories demonstrate the principles in this book—that uncoordinated, unimodal care, especially excessive surgeries, injections and opioids—seldom helps chronic pain patients and often makes them worse.

I have been privileged to know, treat, and learn from many chronic pain patients who were able to manage and surmount their pain through the guidance, encouragement and education of clinicians in a multidisciplinary model. Some of my patients have balked at my edict that they titrate off all opioid pain medication before I treat them—but soon they discover the pain medications were not helping them anyway and start to improve. It is their journeys, some miraculous, that have convinced me over the years that addressing pain from a symptom-oriented biomedical model seldom helps pain patients in the long run.

Such treatment, which has become the contemporary norm despite its expense and lack of evidence base, lacks an appreciation for the many biopsychosocial factors that influence chronic pain like fear, resentment and feelings of being wronged.

It is also clear from these stories that most chronic pain patients begin to recover when they enact two psychological switches—they accept that their pain will never completely go away, that there is no "cure," and they decide to become an active partner in their care rather than a passive recipient.

The first story, Michael's, is a composite of many young men whose on-the-job injuries were mismanaged, causing the patients unnecessary disability and frequently costing them their vocation.

Michael: Portrait of a Back Injury

Michael's life was not supposed to end up like this. After graduating from high school, he joined the local construction union eventually becoming a union steward. His coworkers and employer respected him. He was skilled, knowledgeable, and

© Springer International Publishing Switzerland 2015
S. Vasudevan, *Multidisciplinary Management of Chronic Pain*,
DOI 10.1007/978-3-319-20322-5_11

exceedingly careful in how he performed his job. His salary was good and, combined with his wife's income as a nursing assistant, they could afford a nice home and savings to send their children to college.

All these dreams came to an end when a scaffold Michael was standing on at a construction site collapsed. Michael came tumbling down and found himself on the ground, having trouble getting up. A sharp searing pain began in his back, shooting into his right buttock and coworkers had to help him get up. Though Michael suspected he was not "okay," his first response to the accident was to make sure coworkers were unhurt and to report the incident and injuries to his employer. He brushed his own pain aside—at first.

When Michael got home, his back was stiff and he was limping because of his difficulty in putting weight on his right leg. The next day, his whole body was tight and sore and he even had difficulty getting out of his bed. Still, Michael drove his truck to work and tried to resume his duties until his supervisor, noting his clear pain and distress, suggested Michael leave work and go to a local occupational injury clinic.

At the clinic, Michael was relieved to hear the X-rays showed nothing broken and his intense pain was "muscle strain." He was given medications, including Vicodin and told he would get better in a few weeks. When Michael questioned being given an opioid, having read about their dangers, he was assured it was an appropriate medication for what had happened to him.

After 3 weeks off from work, Michael was no better and was actually getting worse. His lower back pain was becoming more intense and shooting into his right buttock and calf. His toes were tingling. "Rest" from work had not helped at all. He described his pain like "a poker being driven from my back into my toes," a common metaphor pain patients use.

At his follow-up visit at the occupational injury clinic, a physician ordered an MRI scan of the injured area. Now Michael was told he had a "herniated disk and a pinched nerve"—a condition he had heard of in coworkers. The problem was— most of those workers had not returned to work after surgery for those conditions so Michael became concerned. Luckily, the clinic physician said Michael only needed a cortisone injection, not surgery.

Most clinicians who work with chronic pain patients can guess what happened next. After three epidurals, a week apart, there was no improvement in Michael's pain. In fact, after the second epidural, Michael's back pain increased and he developed headaches, which he never had previously. Although, Workers' Compensation insurance paid the medical bills and a small portion of Michael's salary, he was feeling the economic "hit" from the accident and subsequent disability. At his request, clinic doctor cleared him to return to light duty at work but to Michael's disappointment, his employer said none was available.

Six weeks after the scaffold collapsed, Michael's entire lifestyle had changed. Instead of rising at 5 AM, he lay in bed till until at least 9 o'clock, sometimes later. Sleep had become fitful and erratic. He no longer watched what he ate and "consoled" himself with pints of ice cream. Michael no longer played with his children or went out with the family. He was becoming irritable. His family, after showing sympathy for him at first and helping him with services and his responsibilities, now gave him wide berth. Michael felt isolated and misunderstood. He missed work and his coworkers with whom who he used to socialize after work.

On Michael's next visit to the occupational injury clinic, he got a big surprise. A surgeon told him, on the basis of his MRI, he needed surgery to remove the "protruding" disk. Heartened that perhaps they were going to get to the bottom of his pain, Michael scheduled the surgery. Even though the surgery was supposed to be for "disk removal," Michael was asked to sign a consent form for a fusion surgery if the surgeon decided it was needed during the procedure.

Sure enough, when Michael woke up after surgery, he was told the level below the removed disk had been "worn down" and a fusion was installed replete with plates, screws, and artificial bone. The procedure was not only a lot more complicated than he had expected, it was a lot more expensive and his healing time would be greatly elongated.

Now, Michael was put on oxycodone and told to take one to two tablets as needed. Not a "pill person," Michael nevertheless took four to six pills daily for the pain which was extreme. After 4 weeks, when he was released to begin physical therapy, such as riding a stationary bicycle, Michael was shocked and dismayed to find his pain dramatically worsened. What was going on? Michael's low back pain had expanded to his entire back. Toileting and lying in bed were difficult. He began to sleep in a recliner chair away from his wife.

After 6 weeks of continued pain, Michael's OxyContin was bumped up to 10 mg BID. At first, the dose increase helped him participate in his daily physical therapy—which is widely seen as the only defensible use of non-short-term opioids in chronic pain. But soon his back and leg pain increased with a concomitant constant tingling and the sensation of "bugs crawling" on his leg.

What was the response of the clinic's staff to Michael's continued pain? His OxyContin dose was increased to 20 mg BID and he was told to take his Percocet prescription 4–6 day if needed as well. There was more confusion for Michael, too: he was assured that, on the basis of X-rays, his surgery was healing well. Two months after his disk surgery which had turned into a fusion, Michael's surgeon assured him there was no anatomical reason for his pain and referred him to a well-known pain clinic.

More Treatment; Less Pain Relief

At the pain clinic, Michael's pain was attributed to "scar tissue built up" and he was given a series of epidurals and facet injections which provided very short-term relief. Because the relief was only short-lived, Michael was advised to undergo two sets of ablations, or nerve burns, on either side of his body, which paradoxically produced a constant burning sensation. Amazingly, Michael's OxyContin was now increased to 40 mg TID as surgery, injections and ablation had failed in rapid succession.

Meanwhile, things were getting worse at home. Michael's mood and family life continued to degenerate and the man who had led union construction crews he became a grouchy and overweight "coach potato," out of shape and out of sorts.

To its credit, Michael's pain clinic then prescribed a "work hardening" program designed to prepare workers for re-entry into jobs. But clinic staff also added additional medications to his already strong drug regimen including Lyrica, an antiseizure medication, the antidepressant Prozac and Ambien, a sleeping pill sometimes associated with bizarre behavior and psychiatric reactions.

Despite taking OxyContin 40 mg TID a day, Percocet six to eight times a day, Lyrica, Prozac and Ambien, Michael's pain was not improving but worsening—a paradoxical situation I have seen with many chronic pain patients who have been put on high doses of drugs. Soon, to try to relieve his pain and get some sleep, Michael was adding a shot or two of whiskey to his drug cocktail despite warnings on his medication bottles about mixing alcohol with the drugs. Michael had never used illegal drugs or even drank before but 1 day, when an old construction buddy offered him marijuana, he tried it and quickly became habituated to it. The marijuana produced a welcome and rare sense of calm and relief from pain that he had not experienced since the accident.

Unfortunately, smoking marijuana proved to be the beginning of Michael's downfall. Like most pain clinics, Michael had been asked to sign a "narcotic agreement" to only procure medications from medical staff at the clinic. Thanks to the marijuana he was now in violation of his contract. Abruptly and without hearing Michael's explanation, clinic staff discharged Michael with only 1 month supply of OxyContin. What should he do now, he asked the staff? Return to your original surgeon or find another pain clinic, he was told.

Michael did see his surgeon who maintained the X-rays looked fine and no more surgery was in order. When Michael returned for a follow-up visit, the surgeon dismissed him—telling him there was nothing more that could be done and he did not wish to see him again. Michael contacted other pain clinics but because they had access to his first pain clinic records they would not accept him. Michael then called the occupational health clinic where he had gone after the accident for help and they maintained he had been discharged to the care of the surgeon and they could not help him further.

In the meantime, Michael's Workers' Compensation payments ceased. His truck, of which he was so proud, was slated to be repossessed and his house payments were becoming a challenge. His wife, who had been forced to take an extra part-time job was sharing the economic stress; his children barely spoke to him. He stayed up late at night switching television channels, napping only for short times during the day and growing more desperate and despondent. Where had he gone wrong? How could this be happening?

As anyone could have predicted, when Michael used his last OxyContin, he began to develop withdrawal symptoms such as profuse sweating, shivering and loose stools. Frightened, he called a hospital emergency room and was told what he was experiencing was opioid withdrawal. Michael's wife, as concerned as he was, drove him to the hospital emergency room where he was given 20 Vicodin pills to tide him over with no follow-up appointments or treatments or even advice.

Michael did not know what he was more afraid of: the withdrawal symptoms he was experiencing from his weeks on opioid drugs or a return of his excruciating pain—though in all truthfulness, even with his high drug doses, it had not subsided. His identity as a father, husband, and breadwinner was evaporating. While a "take-charge" person who had supervised others on the construction site, he had done nothing but passively accept medical treatments for his pain for months and seldom even asked questions. He and his wife had originally tried to discern whose "fault" his pain odyssey was—doctors, surgeons, clinics—but now he was beyond being angry. Instead he could only think of calling his pastor or his friend who had given him the marijuana. He chose the latter, but this time has asked for "oxys."

Soon Michael and his buddy were on the wrong side of town trying to buy illegal drugs. Since they were new faces in the "hood," most people on the street would not talk to them or help them, thinking they were undercover police. Finally, however they were steered to an alley where they were instructed to put the money through a hole in the door and await their drugs. But as a package appeared through the hole and Michael pocketed it, a squad car appeared with its siren running and Michael was swiftly handcuffed and arrested.

A law-abiding and even "square" person who did not drink, use drugs or even exceed the speed limit, Michael was now in a holding tank with petty thieves and hardened criminals. When allowed one phone call while awaiting arraignment, he called his wife who was as shocked, confused, and terrified as he was.

Luckily for Michael when he went before a night judge, because it was his first offense he was released on a small bond and assigned a court date. He was also remanded to a 7-day drug detoxification program that was publicly funded and did require money Michael no longer had.

Despite his remorse, regret and self-hatred at what his life had become, Michael was nevertheless surprised that after 1 week in the detoxification program his withdrawal symptoms actually went away. In fact, in 1 week of no narcotics, his back and leg pain began to feel better. Michael was not the first, and certainly not the last person habituated to opioids for pain *who discovers the opioids are worsening the pain*. Many of my patients have reported the paradox that the drugs they thought were the solution were the problem.

After his arrest, Michael's marriage hit a rock bottom. His wife was already feeling abused and exploited as she tried to hold the family together through Michael's ordeal. Michael's arrest for illegal drugs was her last straw and she took the children and left for 2 weeks. But after a while, she began to see a change in Michael.

With a mind free from narcotics and sleeping pills, he began to read every book he could about chronic pain and quickly learned about the psychological factors that made pain more than a biomedical phenomenon. He learned how emotional components magnified his pain and adopted mental relaxation techniques including positive thinking, mind-body approaches and self-massage to address pain. Just as importantly, Michael reentered physical therapy with his new attitude and free from drugs. With the help of an exercise therapist and daily workouts on a stationary bicycle, Michael regained his strength and flexibility. Over a period of time, Michael lost his excess 20 pounds and went off the antidepressant which had been the last of his medication.

Like other chronic pain patients who have been on long and discouraging pain odyssey, Michael's life turned around by hitting rock bottom. When things could get no worse—he was in a jail lockup as the common criminal he had become—he grasped at a new attitude and became "teachable." He was willing to learn new ways of dealing with his long-term chronic pain and he embraced the education-based treatment of multidisciplinary care.

While Michael knew he would never return to construction work again, he began to study Computer Assisted Design, applying his knowledge to a relatively new, high-tech field that promised new vocational opportunities and a return to financial solvency.

Like many chronic pain patients, Michael's pain did not fully subside. He did not return to the way he was before the accident but he had a new attitude toward pain of acceptance and positivism. Aware that some days he may still have pain, Michael now had many physical and psychological coping methods he never had previously and understood the concepts of self-management and self-efficacy. More importantly, Michael no longer thought of himself as "poor me." After all he had survived, he knew he was lucky.

Susie's Story

Susie was a successful, 40-year-old executive who worked as deputy director for a large, not-for-profit organization. She was happily married with two children 8 and 6. In her mid-30s, Susie had begun to feel exhausted at times and attributed it to stress and overwork. The symptoms did not go away, however, and she soon began to wake up with pain—sometimes in her neck, other times in her lower back, elbows, or knees.

Suspecting "arthritis," which ran in her family, Susie saw a gynecologist who gave her a clean bill of health and suggested that antianxiety medications might help.

Six months later, despite her medications, Susie was still exhausted and experiencing frequent pain in her neck, shoulders, low back and having headaches. She was becoming irritable at work and at home and her husband suggested she see his internist.

After a scare in which the internist first surmised that Susie was developing rheumatoid arthritis, Susie was reassured that there was "nothing wrong" with her. But Susie's pain and fatigue continued and she began to have trouble falling sleeping in addition to waking up with pain. She and her husband tried different mattresses including the "Sleep Number Bed" she heard advertised so often on TV to no avail. Susie's sleep pattern, constant pain, and fatigue grew worse and her coworkers began to notice it. Reluctantly, on the suggestion of her husband and family members, Susie agreed to see a psychiatrist about the symptoms. After a few visits, she was told there was "no emotional basis to the pain." It was both a relief and not a relief.

Finally, Susie visited a rheumatologist who diagnosed Susie with fibromyalgia as well as with arthritis in her neck. It was a mixed "blessing." Susie was glad to know there was definitely something "wrong"—it was not her imagination or emotions—but, as Susie told me ruefully, "the doctor told me there is no treatment for fibromyalgia and I just had to live with it."

Susie was angry and demoralized. Her life was becoming smaller all the time. She and her husband had given up their family bike rides and she had stopped serving as a judge at children's sports activities and other community events. Susie did not want to go on long trips because of the discomfort of car travel and sleeping in different hotel rooms. Her husband was becoming more irritable as Susie withdrew from the family and life.

Susie's sleep began to degenerate further and she began to miss work. Her employer began to question her motivation and insinuate she had stress at home or was losing her spark and edge or even becoming lazy. This charge was infuriating and shameful to her.

Susie tried a fibromyalgia support group but she felt the participants sounded angry and were more depressed and disabled than she was. For example, group members often discussed a mental cloudiness that they called "Fibrofog" which she had never experienced. After the meetings, she felt worse.

Luckily, Susie found a multidisciplinary pain program not far from where she lived and her improvement began right away. Over the next several weeks she learned that while fibromyalgia was not a progressive, disabling condition and did not affect her bones, joints, nerves, or disks, it was a "syndrome" that would continue to cause aches and pains at different times, sleep difficulties, fatigue, and irritability.

From the multidisciplinary program's physical and occupational therapists she learned to change abnormal postures that were causing her trouble. From a psychologist she got in touch with her frustration over the demands of the many roles she played at home, socially and at work and realized she had to make adjustments.

Soon she was able to engage in appropriate assertive communication with her employer, her family, and her spouse and organize her life differently. Susie began to take time for herself. Her aches and pains became less frequent but when they flared up, she had the education and knowledge to know what to do. From the physical and occupational therapists she learned to avoid doing activities simultaneously without taking breaks and the concept of "pacing."

Today Susie has a more balanced life. She is not free from fibromyalgia symptoms but she has tools to manage them learned from multidisciplinary rehabilitation. And while her "Sleep Number" bed did not fix her pain, she sleeps better in it.

Jeff's Story

At the time of his injury, Jeff, 40, a chiropractor, was working on an elderly patient who began to slip off the table. Stepping around the table to stop the fall, Jeff says he "felt like a piece of Velcro" had pulled in his back. It was the start of a long journey of pain, frustration, and confusion.

During the first month after the injury, walking had not become painful—yet—but sleep was nearly impossible. Jeff had to keep repositioning himself from the constant "achy" pain and could only sleep from 20 min to 2 h a night.

Finally, Jeff consulted an orthopedic surgeon and was told he had disk herniation which required a microdiscectomy. After the surgery, Jeff's pain greatly increased and his physician conducted tests to ensure he had not developed a blood clot. When the pain did not subside, Jeff was back in surgery because, according to the surgeon, "we didn't get all the disk out and it reherniated."

After the second surgery, Jeff's pain persisted and worsened, mostly localizing in his left leg "which felt like it was on fire." His surgeon then referred Jeff to a pain clinic where he received a series of spinal injections and prescriptions for oxycodone and hydrocodone.

Increasingly bedridden, Jeff consulted another surgeon who recommended a spinal fusion after the first two failed surgeries. Because of his chiropractic training, Jeff said he knew that fusion could be effective and he consented. While the fusion operation did have the effect of stabilizing him—"I no longer felt like I was going to fall over," he says—his leg pain did not improve.

Next Jeff consulted a pain specialist who added benzodiazepines, antiseizure drugs, and antidepressants to his opioid prescriptions. Not surprisingly, the drug cocktail had mental effects which affected Jeff's cognition and memory. "My career was slipping away," he says.

As Jeff's pain did not abate, a spinal cord stimulator (SCS) was surgically implanted—an expensive therapy that is not appropriate for all pain patients. While the SCS did interrupt pain signals, says Jeff, "every time I moved I got zapped with a jolt."

Finally, Jeff's Workers' Compensation nurse sent him to our pain center which has a strong multidisciplinary rehabilitation pain program that emphasizes patient education and empowerment. It was at our center that Jeff received the diagnosis of Complex Regional Pain Syndrome (CRPS), discussed in depth in Chap. 10. When I asked Jeff what he thought of his treatment so far and how he should proceed he was aghast. "No one has ever asked *my* opinion on this," he said, "even though I am the one living with the pain."

Once the reason for his pain that was not responsive to any treatments was demystified, Jeff accepted responsibility for his care instead of passively relying on others to fix him and became a partner in his own treatment. In addition to partaking in physical and occupational therapy programs 5 days a week, Jeff began working with a nutritionist, a social worker and a psychologist and his health, attitude, and family life began to improve. As Jeff's pain receded, he was able to stop using the scooter he had relied upon since his first surgery and walk on his own again. He was no longer afraid to bend over to put on his shoes for fear of instigating pain. His fog cleared because he was off the pills. "I became clear-headed again after a long time," says Jeff.

Commensurate with taking responsibility for his own care, Jeff renounced foods he believed made his pain worse through inflammation. After almost 2 years, he got to know his family again. "During the pain nightmare, I wasn't me," he says. "I didn't take the kids to the park; I did not drive them places they needed to go. They did not have a dad." Today, Jeff still can have pain flare-ups but they do not keep him from a rewarding new life which includes a new career as a health educator. Jeff is especially qualified to teach others about chronic pain after his ordeal.

Chapter 12
Conclusion

In this book we have looked at the many factors that complicate the treatment of chronic pain in the United States from the popularity of treatments with questionable or controversial evidence to disability systems that do not encourage functional improvements. Many biopsychosocial factors also affect chronic pain in patients from fear and resentment to anger and feelings of being wronged or a victim.

These confounding factors, as seen in Table 12.1, include:

1. The patient's psychological, social, vocational, and legal milieu
2. Pain enabling behavior of family and clinicians
3. Uncoordinated, unimodal treatment, especially opioids. Injections/interventional approaches and repeated surgeries
4. Disability systems that reward dysfunction
5. Lack of multidisciplinary pain programs and a multidisciplinary approach

Despite the popularity and favorable reimbursement patterns of unimodal and uncoordinated treatment, it is clear in the literature and evidence-based studies that repeated surgeries and injections, long-term use of narcotics are *increasing* and not reducing the number of people who suffer from chronic pain.

We know from countless patient cases that rest, excessive time off from work, excessive focus on pain, and the attitude of "poor me" are "yellow flags" or predictors of continual disability and undesirable pain outcomes in chronic pain patients. Sadly, many patients have been told to abstain from work, their usual activities and to rely on medications—which will not improve their chronic pain but will add to their "disability conviction."

Conversely, it is clear that a multidisciplinary approach to pain rehabilitation that addresses mind, body, social, and behavioral issues shows positive outcomes. The treatment focuses on the patient's return to function not relief of pain and seeks to induce a change in the patient's attitude toward pain as we see in Table 12.2. These positive outcomes are evident whether they are quantified in pain and quality of life, healthcare costs or a patient's dependency on drugs and the healthcare system, as we as we saw in Chap. 8.

© Springer International Publishing Switzerland 2015
S. Vasudevan, *Multidisciplinary Management of Chronic Pain*,
DOI 10.1007/978-3-319-20322-5_12

Table 12.1 Factors which complicate chronic pain in patients

Influences on patient	Psychological, social, vocational, legal
Enabling of pain behaviors	Family, clinicians
Uncoordinated pain treatment	Excessive surgeries, injections, opioids
Disability/compensation systems	Can reward dysfunction
Lack of multidisciplinary care	Few programs; little awareness

Table 12.2 Keys to patient recovery from pain

Resume activities as soon as possible
Participate in care and treatment decisions
Accept that pain will not completely be eliminated
Avoid self-pity and develop positive attitude

It is likely that as "accountable" health plans develop in the United States, pegged to total and lifetime costs of conditions and diseases and not short-term "snapshots," the value of multidisciplinary programs in pain rehabilitation will be newly appreciated and their availability restored. Even as multidisciplinary pain programs have all but vanished in the United States, they are growing in much of the rest of the world for the simple reason that *they work*.

For example, as we saw in Chap. 9, a "back attack" should be a wake-up call and an occasion to reeducate a patient about his health status and lifestyle. While a back attack may not appear as serious as a cardiovascular event, its effect on the patient's quality of life and dependence on the healthcare system are similar. That is why the COST B13 Working Group established "European guidelines for the management of chronic nonspecific low back pain" (AACVPR 2015; Airaksinen et al. 2006) similar to American Association of Cardiovascular and Pulmonary Rehabilitation (AACVPR) guidelines which recognize the importance of physical, psychological, and social changes in reducing death and disability from a heart attack.

Multidisciplinary treatment is especially effective in helping patients change their "pain behaviors" which have been recognized as factors that increase the patient's pain and disability conviction. Certainly it is natural for medical professionals to respond to a patient's pain with empathy, sympathy, and the provision of medications. Employers and insurers often respond with granting the patient time off from work and financial settlements and family members often excuse the patient from his responsibilities.

But, as any parent can tell you, behaviors that are "rewarded" in this fashion will become more frequent or "reinforced." Behavior that is ignored or negatively reinforced will tend to disappear. In keeping with such principles of behavioral modification, multidisciplinary pain treatment focuses on "behavioral shaping"—rewarding well behaviors such as active participation in therapies and a positive attitude and ignoring sick behaviors whether drug seeking or excessive physical displays of pain.

In countries where certain diseases/conditions are not highly rewarded by compensation, such as from automobile injuries, claims of harm are seen to be less. In other situations where there is significant litigation and potential for financial reward, claims of injury and pain increase.

A Movie Addresses Chronic Pain

In 2014, a movie was released in the United States which showed both the relentless daily emotional and physical toll of chronic pain and the switches in emotions and attitude that often precede a patient improving.

The movie, *Cake*, starred actress Jennifer Aniston who plays a well-to-do California lawyer suffering from chronic pain, the cause of which viewers do not know. Claire is so wracked with pain she cannot even sit up in the car. Her housekeeper, Silvana, drives her to the doctors and other places she needs to go while she reclines in the car.

Like so many real chronic pain patients recovering from car and work accidents or living with pain that has no clear cause, Claire has become addicted to opioids and her entire life revolves around getting drugs and hiding her addicted state from others. One scene shows how she manipulates and charms a doctor into writing a prescription that does not have authorization; another scene follows Claire and her housekeeper Silvana as they drive all the way to Tijuana to procure Claire's drugs which she then hides in a statue as they cross back into the United States.

One of the definitions of addiction is pursuit and use of a needed substance *regardless of unwanted consequences* and Claire and Silvana's Tijuana foray is a case in point: they are stopped by the authorities for the opioids they are trying to smuggle in and only because Claire's husband, from whom she has become estranged, is a government official do they escape prosecution and/or jail.

Anyone who has had chronic pain or treated it will recognize Claire's cluster of psychological and behavioral responses to her condition that make her pain worse not better: overriding focus on the pain, a narrowing life and isolation, "pain behaviors" that are rewarded by others and a feeling of being an innocent victim who has been wronged.

Cake also demonstrates a treatment precept we have stressed repeatedly in this book: long-term opioid treatment for chronic pain is almost never indicated; it will not relieve pain on a long-term basis and can worsen a patient's pain through opioid-induced hyperalgesia. In treating chronic pain patients, opioid therapy is only valuable when used to help a patient participate in the therapies, especially physical therapy, that address the pain—and not to just cover it up, as we discussed in Chap. 6. Claire's downward spiral on long-term opioids, both worsening her pain and her mental state, are clearly portrayed.

At the beginning of the movie, Claire does not identify with others in a chronic pain support group and unleashes sarcastic remarks that get her banned from the group. She embraces fear, remains in isolation and takes her anger out against others. However, later in the movie, viewers became aware that it is not just physical pain but emotional pain that is driving Claire's suffering. Once she is able to get "in touch" with the emotions behind her pain, her anger begins to dissipate.

Following the suicide of another woman in the chronic pain group—which is replayed through flashbacks and dreams—Claire befriends the widower husband who is now raising the son alone. By spending time with the husband and son, Claire comes to get "out of herself" as she symbolically fills the place of the lost mother and wife. She sees she has something to offer, loses her self-focus, and "reframes" her pain.

Toward the end of the movie, Claire gets another "lesson" in the existence of others' pain besides her own. Her housekeeper, Silvana, loses her temper at Claire's self-centered self-pity after having to save Claire from a suicide attempt in which she lies down on train tracks. You "treat me like a dog" and "pay me like a dog," too screams Silvana in Spanish, though it is not clear that Claire understands the language. The tirade seems to be a wake-up call to Claire.

Families and friends of patients with chronic pain will no doubt relate to Silvana's outburst from spending months or even years exhibiting patience and compassion to increasingly irascible pain sufferers. Strained family relations are a hallmark of chronic pain conditions—yet they change for the better when patients adopt newer attitudes.

Cake's dramatic conclusion in which Claire finds new meaning in her life after wishing for death clearly shows the power of *acceptance* in chronic pain patients. Toward the end of the movie, Claire allows herself to feel the emotions she has been covering up with opioids. Most recovery programs whether for addiction or previous trauma focus on processing unpleasant emotions rather than "pushing them down."

Several scenes in *Cake* also demonstrate the "hurt versus harm" dichotomy that we have stressed in this book. Claire predictably clashes with her physical therapist over her unwillingness to do exercises that hurt her in the short-term even though they will help her in the long run. But, in the last scene in the movie, Claire signals that she is willing to endure the "hurt" to recover from pain. She enacts an effort-filled and successful attempt to finally *sit up* in the car for this first time. It serves as a visual metaphor for her resolution to face her pain, reframe it and not let it control her life.

The Power of Acceptance

> The Most Profound Choice In Life is Either Accept the Things As They are or to Accept the Responsibility For Changing Them

In Chap. 2, we looked at the book *The Promise*: *Never Have Another Negative Thought Again* by Graham Price (Pearson 2013) which chronicles this acceptance process—a phenomenon that Price calls "pacceptance" (for positive acceptance) that is, arguably, the single biggest predictor of improvement in chronic pain patients. The process of acceptance is often linked to the patients' realization that their pain and the events that caused it cannot be undone and will not go away.

Many patients believe that there is, or *should be*, a magic pill or procedure to take away their chronic pain and are disappointed to hear that we can't "cure" it—though we can help them manage it well. We medical professionals share their disappointment.

When patients finally accept that their pain cannot be "cured," it can be a bittersweet moment in which they surrender both their dreams and their battle and wave the white flag. In 12-Step recovery programs from addiction, this is the moment when a person has hit a "bottom" and is "sick and tired of being sick and tired." This moment of "enough" causes a shift in perspective in which a patient often reframes his situation and becomes willing to try a new attitude and a new path for the first time. Often patients also accept at this point that their pain and situation are *no one's particular "fault"*—whether an employer, doctor, motorist, or surgeon. Renouncing anger, resentment, remorse, and even anger at themselves greatly help patients control their pain as we explored in previous chapters.

After hitting a "bottom" in which they admit they are powerless over their chronic pain, patients often become open-minded and "come to believe" that a new and different treatment path could work. They proceed to place their trust in a multidisciplinary approach or their physical therapist and psychologist for the first time—despite their doubts that the recommendations of these clinicians will work. In a sense, patients have become so frustrated and discouraged with their current path, they have become open-minded and "teachable."

There is another change that occurs when pain patients undergo this acceptance process: they became active participants in their pain rehabilitation. Most current unimodal pain treatment reduces patients to passively taking a pill or submitting to injections or surgery; with a new, acceptant attitude, a patient now partners with his clinicians—actively working his treatments. Exhorting patients to act as their own "healer" (in conjunction with other medical professionals) can be disarming to patients because it is at variance with much current medical practice. But self-management, self-efficacy, and self-care are the foundation of the multidisciplinary approach to chronic pain—and why it works so well.

It is often said, "Your attitude determines your altitude" and those of us who work in pain rehabilitation know it is true. When pain patients undergo the acceptance process, it lets them harness and redirect anger and sadness, possibly for the first time. They are now free to apply it toward positive goals and experience motivation to improve and rebuild their lives. This is the point, many patients tell me, where they decide they are no longer going to be "controlled" by the pain but are going to control *it*. I have seen this process in my patients and it often precedes their resolve to get better.

Patients must be willing to get rid of the life they had planned to live the life that is waiting for them.

This moment of surrender often changes the field and ground for these patients. Just as people with chronic alcoholism have been known to say, "I had to quit because I couldn't stop," pain patients might say, "I had to accept my pain because I couldn't live with it." It is a paradox but it is also a true turning point.

When pain patients cease their fight and regard their pain as something they have to accept, they often become newly motivated to learn different ways of dealing with their pain. With the help of occupational and physical therapists, patients learn how to avoid putting excessive strain on their body as they gradually increase activity levels. They become more independent and self-confident at home, work, and in other activities as they learn new tools and develop self-efficacy. I recount some of my patients' success stories in Chap. 11, Patient Profiles.

The Power of Attitude

Recently, I saw a wounded veteran from the Afghanistan war interviewed on television. "I don't want my life to be about my injury," he told the newscaster. "I want it to be about my life *after the injury*." The soldier observed that all the veterans he knows who have overcome significant injuries have positive spirits and positive attitudes. The scores of runners and bystanders who were injured in the Boston Marathon bombings in 2013 expressed similar philosophies of focusing on the positive, despite their many injuries. Even though some of the victims were likely to never run again, those who had positive attitudes were already focusing on sports that they *could* participate in.

Some patients have significant disease but give little verbal and nonverbal expression of their pain as pain behaviors. Others, including those with fibromyalgia, migraine headaches or even fatigue often think of themselves as completely disabled. Social modeling, belief systems, individual and family histories and different cultures explain the great variation in pain expression but a unifying principle in effective coping with pain and disability is *attitude*. A good example is Nick Vujicic, a motivational speaker from Australia who is missing all four limbs from tetra-amelia syndrome but who refuses to think of himself as disabled.

In my previous book, *Pain: A Four-Letter Word You Can Live With* (1995), I examined the many four-letter words that insinuate their way into the thought patterns of chronic pain patients such as rage, fear, can't, hurt, loss and of course pain. I stress that patients can substitute positive four-letter words like hope, life, pace and love to cultivate a more optimistic attitude, especially when working with multidisciplinary professionals who address their physical and mental needs. They can also substitute work, team, live and even "gate" from what they have learned about the Gate Theory and how they can dampen their pain.

I also urge patients to embrace the four-letter word *read* and study pain in the many books available for laypeople. Discovering the complexity of pain and its many "faces" as well as how millions cope, enlarges patients' view so that they no longer think they are somehow unique or personally "cursed" with a pain condition.

For this reason, self-help groups for pain patients, often affiliated with pain treatment centers, also work well.

Many patients have also shared that their ability to pray is an important part of their recovery and control over pain—another useful four-letter word. The role of spirituality in pain management is important. Certainly before the "scientific era" of the 1600s, pain was regarded almost exclusively in a spiritual and religious context. As knowledge about mind/body connections grows, we begin to see how psychology, medicine, philosophy, and spirituality intermingle. A good example is the popularity of the book, *Proof of Heaven*, by neurosurgeon Eben Alexander who notes that while he was in a coma for 7 days, he was able to visit "the other life" (2012).

In an intriguing book titled *Ask and it Shall Be Given: Learning to Manifest Your Desires* (Hicks and Hicks 2004) Esther and Jerry Hicks explore the untapped power of positive thought which, they write, can change someone's belief system and even circumstances. Negative emotions and the negative energy they create can actually "attract" negative experiences say the authors.

As we have discussed in other chapters, the belief system of a chronic pain patient influences his behavior which in turn influences his pain and often loops back and reinforces his belief system and his disability conviction. That is why I urge clinicians to balance disturbing diagnoses like failed back surgery syndrome or disk "problems at every level" with positive findings about what is *right* with a patient.

Other authors such as Wayne Dyer confirm that people can shape their own thoughts despite lifelong self-defeating thinking and old, fixed programming. While habitual behavior whether eating, smoking, or responses to chronic pain is frequently viewed as immutable and a result of genes, prompting patients to say "I can't change who I am," people can indeed change says Dr. Dyer, citing numerous scientific studies. Dr. Dyer also believes that the spirit and the mind are more capable of effecting change than the ego and the body.

Bruce Lipton, author of the *Biology of Belief*, reaches similar conclusions about the ability of one's belief system to actually affect biological functions (Lipton 2008). In one example cited in his book, two sets of hotel maid did identical work but one group was told they were doing "exercises." At the end of an 8-week period, the maids who believed they were involved in positive activity and "exercising" showed superior measurements of cardiovascular fitness than the "control" group who thought they were simply doing their job.

Effective Communication with the Chronic Pain Patient

When you first see a chronic pain patient, he often has been in the healthcare system for quite a while and received many treatments which he believes have not been successful. He may have been told he had a muscle strain—but it did not get better. Perhaps he received injections and they didn't help. The patient likely received surgery which did not meet expectations and even led to more pain. The patient was also probably told that medication would help only to experience side effects and continued pain. To add insult to injury, the patient often suspects his pain is not believed to exist—that he is thought to be exaggerating. No wonder pain patients are often frustrated with their physicians.

Some physicians when they begin to conclude that they cannot help or comfort a patient will pull away, leaving patients feeling abandoned. We do not like failure and when our best efforts fail it can feel like a reflection on us. In my experience, if the patient and medical professionals are patient, however, both will see improvements with a multidisciplinary model of treatment.

One of our first challenges as medical professionals with chronic pain patients is to rebuild the lost trust between us. Without trust there is no way to inspire the patient to want to try the new "road" of multidisciplinary pain treatment which will involve elimination of opioids and use of appropriate medication, addressing psychological and emotional issues and educating and empowering the patient about pain and pain management. The success of the first visit rests on effective communication—how well we understand the patient's pain history and how well we can convey the multidisciplinary approach to pain management.

Physicians are not always good listeners and some studies have found we interrupt patients every 18 s. If a patient feels rushed and does not have adequate time to convey his concerns the trust gap widens, so it important we give the patient "listen time."

Despite the fact that I usually have extensive records sent to me, I like to hear patients describe their injuries and pain odyssey in their own words. I ask them to point to the specific locations of their pain and to describe the pain's quality and its intensity on a one-to-ten scale. I also ask whether their pain is associated with any weakness, numbness or tingling and what makes it better or worse. It is also useful to have patients describe in their own words what kind of treatments they have received and what has worked and not worked.

A good way to extract information from your patient is to ask open-ended questions—not "Where is your pain?" but "How can I help?" After you discern a thorough history of their injury, how it happened and their main complaint, it is also useful to inquire about the patient's family. Because a patient's pain both affects his family and is affected by it, I spend a great deal of time finding out how long a patient has been married, whether it is his first or subsequent marriage, how many children there are and how the spouse has responded to the pain situation. Certainly family and financial stresses only add to chronic pain and this line of questioning is a good way to reveal stressors.

Your patient interview should also probe the patient's vocation, hobbies and social activities. Many patients, in addition to being off work, have become isolated and ceased doing things they once enjoyed, adding to their pain focus and discouraged mood.

Four questions that are very useful in understanding your patient and helping you treat the "patient" not the "pain" are found in Table 12.3.

Table 12.3 Four questions to ask a new pain patient	What do you think is causing your pain?
	What you think should be done about your pain?
	What are the things you can no longer do because of pain?
	What do you expect to do if your pain is controlled?

What Do You Think Is Causing Your Pain?

While the patient usually answers, "I don't know. I'm not a doctor," this question can often reveal the patient's belief system and convictions about his pain experience. At first a patient will often repeat something he might have been saying for a long time like, "The accident caused the pain and 4 years later, I am still in pain!" but if you probe, you can often discover other factors that are big influences in the patient's life.

What You Think Should Be Done About the Pain?

This question usually draws the same answer as the first one and can even draw anger. Patients are often angry that surgery, injections, other interventions and physical therapy have not "worked." They convey they are becoming, hopeless, frustrated and at the end of their rope and that they believe nobody can help them. These emotions grow out of a passive model of a healthcare system that "fixes" pain and can lead a patient to consider a participatory model.

What Are the Things You Can No Longer Do Because of Your Pain?

This question can inspire a patient to say "I can't do anything anymore" but it often opens the gateway to finding out what values and activities have made a patient's life meaningful up until now and "who the patient is." Is the patient missing an activity, using a skill, pursuing an interest or an important relationship that has changed? This question will often tease the information out.

What Do You Expect to Do If We Can Get Your Pain Under Control?

This question will help you spare your patients unrealistic expectations and disappointments. For example, a 45-year-old man who has had three back surgeries and is 30 or more pounds overweight will not likely reclaim the physical condition and abilities he had at 20 again. Nor will a reduction in pain symptoms fix a troubled marriage or vocational career. Have them outline the realistic SMART goals they wish to accomplish as discussed in Chap. 8, Creating a Multidisciplinary Team.

These four questions can jolt a patient out of an old way of thinking about his pain and an old way of interacting with medical professionals. A patient of mine who I will call Tom experienced just such a Gestalt. Not yet 40, by the time I saw Tom, he had undergone several unsuccessful back surgeries, two unsuccessful ablations, countless epidural injections for pain and implantation of a spinal cord stimulator. He was taking high doses of OxyContin and Percocet as well as the antiseizure drug Lyrica and an antidepressant and sleeping pill. Despite the high dosages of prescription drugs, he was getting worse not better.

After I ascertained Tom's pain narrative and his frustrations in the healthcare system, I looked him in the eye and asked him "what do you want *me* to do about it?" While my confrontational tone might have seemed unsympathetic, I wanted to spark a psychological shift in his thinking. My directness with Tim worked. "Up until now, the doctors kept saying, 'trust us'," Tom told me. "This is the first time the doctor was implying that *I* knew something about my own pain and treatment and that I was a partner in my care."

Accepting responsibility for his pain for the first time instead of relying on physicians to "fix" it, Tom threw himself into physical and occupational therapy programs 5 days a week. He titrated off the drugs and "became clear-headed again after a long time," he told me. Slowly, he began interacting with people again and ending his isolation. He was no longer afraid of activities that he thought would reactivate his pain. Tom is now in a new and rewarding career, his life no longer ruled by pain.

The "Milwaukee" Approach to Counseling Patients with Chronic Pain

Years ago, I developed a method of collecting information from patients that has been invaluable to me and to my colleagues. It is called the Milwaukee Approach as seen in Table 12.4. I presented this initially at a meeting of the International Association for the Study of Pain (IASP) in Hamburg, Germany in 1984. Both my patients and medical professionals I work with find it helpful in setting the stage for optimal communication.

Table 12.4 The "Milwaukee" approach

M	Milieu—create a positive caring environment
I	Information—find out patient's knowledge level about his condition; provide information
L	Label—help patient understand labels or diagnoses he has been given
W	Why—help patient understand why his pain may persist; review the theories
A	Aims—Establish short- and long-term realistic goals with patient
U	Understanding—Make sure the patient understands the new path of pain treatment
K	Knowledge—Explain why pain can exist without clear "cause"; the rationale for multidisciplinary treatment.; why long-term opioids are not helpful
E	Engage—Find out how patient feels about his pain, his life, and his visit
E	End—End visit with a promise to address patient's additional questions; provide hope

Milieu

The environment in which you speak with your patients should be positive, caring, and comfortable. After your examination of the patient, sit down with him and his family members, if they are available, and discuss the findings. Self-disclosure—telling a patient something about yourself, your background and your interest in treating pain—often establishes a closer bond.

Information

It is crucial that you discover what the patient knows and doesn't know about pain in general and his condition in particular. A patient's knowledge level about his condition greatly affects his pain experience and treatment. Provide the patient the information you have gained through review of his records and your examination.

Label

Patients are frequently given labels and diagnoses that confuse and scare them and keep them from complying with appropriate treatment. Taking a few minutes to explain the relevant pain diagnoses to your patients is valuable as well as the *psychological factors that affect chronic pain*, including the role of depression. Explain what is "right" with the patient, and note that "what is wrong" is a small part of their whole person.

Why

Patients usually have questions about why they are continuing to have pain despite the passage of time and seemingly adequate approaches to treatment. This is an opportunity to explain to a patient the difference between acute and chronic pain and review the treatment he has received so far.

Aims

It is important to discuss long- and short-term goals of treatment with your patients. For example, they need to appreciate that chronic pain is seldom, if ever, "cured" but that it can be well managed. Also, the patient should understand that a multidisciplinary approach to chronic pain emphasizes long-term functional improvement rather than short-term relief from pain. Review goals that are SMART (Specific, Measurable, Achievable, Realistic, and Time-based) to achieve, if the patient makes the decision to take responsibility for his care and life.

Understanding

When the visit is coming to a close, try to ascertain that the patient grasps everything that has been discussed and wants to move ahead. Let him know the new path to chronic pain care includes both body and mind treatments and he, as the patient, will be an active participant in the care. Tell them the different theories you reviewed, as needed.

Knowledge

A brief and simple explanation of the major theories of pain (the Gate Theory, Door Bell Theory, earlier in this chapter) gives helps in understanding why pain can persist without a clear "cause." Explain to the patient the rationale of physical and occupational therapies, TENS unit and/or injections if they are part of the plan and why and how a behavioral psychologist who uses Cognitive Behavior Therapy (CBT), Acceptance and Commitment Therapy (ACT) or other approaches of "reframing" their thoughts about pain is helpful. Patients should also understand why long-term use of opioids will worsen and not help their condition and that other useful medications exist.

Engage in Feeling

Many pain patients have strong emotions about their pain, sometimes feeling like medical professionals are not helping them or taking their pain seriously. Probe your patient's feelings about what you have told him during the visit. If he feels frustration that you are not offering a "cure," this is an opportunity for discussion. Take time to address the anger and sadness that are often present. I have often had patients begin weeping during a visit which is an important and useful part of the emotional process.

End

Conclude a visit with a pain patient by leaving the door open for questions that subsequently arise. Encourage the patient to write down any additional questions to discuss at the next appointment. Provide the patient with hope and the expectation of his active participation in the shared decision-making process with the multidisciplinary team.

Conclusion

As this book has emphasized repeatedly, the goal of multidisciplinary care is not to "cure" the patient's pain but to encourage him to learn and practice self-care, self-efficacy, and self-management of his pain. Multidisciplinary treatment provides a "cafeteria" of different approaches like physical therapy, exercises, psychological support, and medication when needed but in the last analysis, it is the *patient's* pain and he is best equipped to deal with it.

Many chronic pain patients when they accept their pain and achieve a new attitude say to me "the pain is no longer controlling me; I am controlling the pain." They describe their ability to live successful lives despite recurrent or chronic pain, sometimes finding new careers and passions and bringing renewed affection to their families. While none would return to their previous battles with chronic pain, many cite unexpected gifts that were received from their ordeal with pain.

> Successful patients are the ones who do not view obstacles as stumbling blocks but as *stepping stones* in their recovery and in regaining control over their pain.

When it comes to overcoming chronic pain, I like to remind patients of the mystery of an acorn or any seed. Seeds have an internal compass that tells them when they have the right moisture, soil nutrients and temperature to sprout, even if they have been dormant for years. Like a seed, if the chronic pain patient does not have the environment he needs, nothing will make him "sprout." And, like the seed, if he has the *correct* growth requirements, usually multidisciplinary rehabilitation, nothing can stop him from sprouting!

Closing Thoughts

As we noted in the introduction of this book, a federal advisory group has released a National Pain Strategy (NPS) which, if implemented, would shift national pain care toward the multidisciplinary and biopsychosocial approaches described in this book.

The underlying principles in the National Pain Strategy Affirm

1. Effective pain management is a moral imperative, a professional responsibility, and the duty of people in the healing professions.
2. Chronic pain can be a disease in itself. Chronic pain has a distinct pathology, causing changes throughout the nervous system that often worsen over time. It has significant psychological and cognitive correlates and can constitute a serious, separate disease entity.
3. *Value of comprehensive treatment.* Pain results from a combination of biological, psychological, and social factors and often requires comprehensive approaches to prevention and management.
4. *Need for interdisciplinary approaches.* Given chronic pain's diverse effects, interdisciplinary assessment and treatment may produce the best results for people with the most severe and persistent pain problems.
5. *Importance of prevention.* Chronic pain has such severe impacts on all aspects of the lives of people who have it that every effort should be made to achieve both primary prevention (e.g., in surgery for broken hip) and secondary prevention (of the transition from the acute to the chronic state) through early intervention.

6. *Wider use of existing knowledge*. While there is much more to be learned about pain and its treatment, even existing knowledge is not always used effectively, and thus substantial numbers of people suffer unnecessarily.
7. *The conundrum of opioids*. The committee recognizes the serious problem of diversion and abuse of opioid drugs, as well as questions about their usefulness long-term, but believes that when opioids are used as prescribed and appropriately monitored, they can be safe and effective, especially for acute, postoperative, and procedural pain, as well as for patients near the end of life who desire more pain relief.
8. Roles for patients and clinicians: The effectiveness of pain treatment depends greatly on the strength of the *clinician–patient relationship*; pain treatment is never about the clinician's intervention alone, but about the clinician and patient (and family) working together.
9. *Value of public health and community-based approach*: Many features of the problem of pain lend themselves to public health approaches—a concern about the large number of people affected, disparities in occurrence and treatment, and the goal of prevention cited above. Public health education can help counter the myths, misunderstandings, stereotypes, and stigma that hinder better care (IPRCC 2015).

The IPRCC report reinforces the principles and philosophy that have guided my own practice and that of my colleagues working in pain medicine for many years and we laud the recommendations.

However, without mechanisms to fund a national shift toward multidisciplinary care and away from the uncoordinated, unimodal care, the report's recommendations will not be meaningful or affect the day-to-day lives of pain patients.

I hope, as I am sure the readers of this book do, that reimbursement steps are taken to make the promise and pain relief of multidisciplinary pain programs available to patients.

References

AACVPR. (2015). Cardiac rehabilitation fast facts. Retrieved from https://www.aacvpr.org/about/aboutcardiacpulmonaryrehab/tabid/560/default.aspx.

Alexander, E. (2012). *Proof of heaven*. New York: Simon and Schuster.

Airaksinen, O., Brox, J. I., Cedraschi, C., Hildebrandt, J., Klaber-Moffett, J., Kovacs, F., et al. (2006). European guidelines for the management of chronic nonspecific low back pain. *European Spine Journal, 15*(Suppl. 2), 192–300.

Hicks, J., & Hicks, E. (2004). *Ask and it shall be given: Learning to manifest your desires*. Carlsbad, CA: Hay House.

Interagency Pain Research Coordinating Committee. (2015). *A comprehensive population health-level strategy for pain: National pain strategy*. Washington, DC: HHS.

Lipton, B. (2008). *The biology of belief: Unleashing the power of consciousness, matter, and miracles*. Carlsbad, CA: Hay House.

Price, G. (2013). *The promise: Never have another negative thought again*. London, England: Pearson Education Limited.

Vasudevan, S. (1995). *Pain: A four-letter word you can live with*. Milwaukee, WI: Montgomery Media.

Index

© Springer International Publishing Switzerland 2015
S. Vasudevan, *Multidisciplinary Management of Chronic Pain,*
DOI 10.1007/978-3-319-20322-5